The Cancer Pain Sourcebook

The Cancer Pain
SOURCEBOOK

Roger S. Cicala, M.D.

Medical Director
Methodist Comprehensive Pain Institute

CB
CONTEMPORARY BOOKS

Library of Congress Cataloging-in-Publication Data

The cancer pain sourcebook / Roger S. Cicala [editor]; contributing
authors, David van Alstine—[et al.].
    p. cm.
Includes bibliographical references and index.
ISBN 0-7373-0423-5
    1. Cancer pain. I. Cicala, Roger S. II. Alstine, David van.

RC262.C291196 2001
616.99'4—dc21

00-053478

Published by Contemporary Books
A division of The McGraw-Hill Companies
4255 West Touhy Avenue, Lincolnwood, Illinois 60712, U.S.A.

01 02 03 04 DHD 18 17 16 15 14 13 12 11 10 9 8 7 6 5 4 3 2 1

International Standard Book Number: 0-7373-0423-5

Interior design by Kate Mueller
Printed and bound by R.R. Donnelley & Sons Co.

Contributing Authors

David van Alstine, M.D.
Interventional Anesthesiology and Pain Management, Methodist Comprehensive Pain Institute; Diplomate in Pain Management, American Board of Anesthesiology; Staff Anesthesiologist, Medical Anesthesia Group, P. C.

Daniel Brookoff, M.D.
Oncology, Internal Medicine, and Pain Management; Associate Medical Director, Methodist Comprehensive Pain Institute; Associate Director, Medical Education, Methodist Healthcare; Clinical Associate Professor, University of Tennessee College of Medicine.

Claudio Andrès Feler, M.D., F.A.C.S.
Functional and Palliative Neurosurgery, Methodist Comprehensive Pain Institute and Semmes-Murphey Clinic; Assistant Professor of Neurosurgery, University of Tennessee College of Medicine.

David Leggett, M.D.
Interventional Anesthesiology and Pain Management, Methodist Comprehensive Pain Institute; Diplomate in Pain Management, American Board of Anesthesiology; Staff Anesthesiologist, Medical Anesthesia Group, P. C.

Contents

Contents

About the Methodist Comprehensive Pain Institute

Traditionally, medical science has considered pain to be a symptom of an underlying disease. Doctors should simply cure the disease to stop the pain. It was obvious, however, that this didn't always work. Some diseases simply couldn't be cured. Over time, in some conditions, pain seemed almost to become a disease itself, causing secondary problems and symptoms. Doctors who treated chronic pain patients often became frustrated as it became apparent they could not offer much help.

Beginning in the 1950s, Dr. John Bonica and others originated the concept of multidisciplinary pain clinics or pain centers. The idea was a simple and logical one in theory: Many different medical and other health care specialists spent a significant part of their time treating pain as a primary condition. If all these different specialists practiced together, they could provide better care for chronic pain patients.

When pain centers worked, they worked well. Unfortunately, putting a simple theory into practice was far more difficult than it sounded. Often, the various specialists in a center had very different ideas; fighting and "turf wars" erupted between the doctors. Financial problems reared their ugly heads, as they so often do. The simple reality was that some of the specialists in a center could make far better livings practicing by themselves than in a group. By the 1980s, many multidisciplinary centers had just one or two different specialists on their staff.

Some excellent pain centers survived and thrived. Most of these, however, were located in university teaching hospitals, which unfortunately are not available to many people. Some of the others were large corporate entities that could hire doctors from various specialties. For some patients, the experience at these centers, while excellent from a medical and technical standpoint, was overwhelming. Three or four different doctors would examine the patient, perform tests, and then meet as a committee behind closed doors to discuss the case. Depending on the treatment plan, the patient might see one or several of the doctors together or at different times.

The idea for the Methodist Comprehensive Pain Institute began in 1996. Several of us, each from a different medical specialty, had arrived at the same conclusion: We wanted to be able to draw on one another's expertise in order to provide better care for our patients, but we didn't want to give up the individual contact with our patients that private practice allowed. At the same time, Methodist Hospital (actually the world's largest private hospital) wanted to offer multidisciplinary care for people with chronic pain. Everyone agreed that there must be a way to accomplish this, while avoiding the problems that others experienced with the "corporate group of physicians" approach.

The solution we've used, the concept of primary pain care doctors, is so simple that we're all still surprised at how well it works. Each patient at The Methodist Comprehensive Pain Institute is initially evaluated by a trained pain specialist who becomes that patient's primary care doctor for pain management. That doctor coordinates the patient's care, involving the other specialists at the institute as needed. These primary care doctors generally work full-time at the institute. The other specialists maintain their own private practices, but see patients at the pain institute at certain times each week.

From a medical perspective, this allows several different specialists to be involved in the patient's care, providing many different options for controlling the patient's pain. From the patient's point of view, there is no "parade of doctors," which can be so overwhelming. Since each specialist comes to the institute, the patient does not have to go to several offices, filling out different forms each time. Even insurance companies benefit, since the primary care physician makes sure only the appropriate doctors are consulted, and tests are not repeated.

The result is that while the institute can provide even the most complex pain management procedures performed by subspecialists using the newest technology, we only do so when absolutely necessary. For many patients, a thorough evaluation to determine the actual causes of pain, followed by simple medication adjustments or other forms of therapy, can provide all the relief they need. For those that do not respond to these initial therapies, more specialized treatments are available. Before such a procedure is considered, however, a primary care doctor, who hasn't invested thousands of dollars in the equipment or spent years training how to use it, must agree that it is the best possible solution.

In these days of mission statements and policy manuals, we believe that a few simple sayings provide the guidelines we follow in order to give the best possible care to a cancer patient in pain:

- *Primum non nocere* (First, do no harm).
- Know that pain is any sensation that is uncomfortable to the patient.
- Do whatever is necessary to relieve the pain, but no more than that, because in medicine, attempting better often ruins good enough. In simpler terms, if it ain't broke, don't fix it.

Acknowledgments

The Methodist Comprehensive Pain Institute could never have started and certainly would never have grown this quickly without support from the administration of Methodist Hospitals of Memphis. Cindy Lekhy's unceasing efforts and enthusiastic support began when the institute was simply an idea and carried us through our opening and first expansion. Maurice Elliott, Gary Shorb, Dave Ramsey, and Robin Barca have given us the support we needed to grow, even when they had to use smoke and mirrors to make the funding appear. More importantly, they've trusted our judgment and let us do what we thought best, even when they weren't quite sure they agreed with us. Our advisory board, Drs. John Duckworth, Irv Fleming, Raz Dilawari, Dennis Higdon, and David Cunningham, has always given wonderful advice, especially during the first years when every decision was critical.

Most of all, we wish to thank the staff of the institute. They are the ones that spend untold hours every day actually taking care of the patients we see for a few minutes. It's hard to remember when the staff consisted only of Ami, Christie, Dana, and Tammy. Over time, Barry, Leavy, Donell, Barbara, Brenda, Rosemary, Shelly, Alicia, Vicky, Stacee, Elsie, and Ginger have joined us. Not to mention Becky, Carol, Karen, and Charlotte, who are always willing to help out. And this still doesn't recognize all the departments in Methodist Hospital, from pharmacy to pastoral care, which have given time, advice, and guidance as we've started one new type of therapy after another.

Introduction

For many years, pain management has been the forgotten stepchild in the family of medical specialties that care for cancer patients. From a medical training standpoint, this makes some sense; the primary goal of medicine is always to cure the disease. Treating the symptom—in this case the pain—is medically somewhat like an admission of failure to achieve the primary goal—cure. Several different medical specialties focus entirely on treating, and hopefully curing, cancer: medical oncology, surgical oncology, and radiation oncology, to name a few. The focus of them all, as it should be, is to cure the patient's cancer.

A patient's first question after receiving a diagnosis of cancer is usually "Can it be cured?" The presence of all these specialists is reassuring; everything possible will be done to cure the disease. The cancer patient's second question, which sometimes doesn't occur for several days, is usually, "Will I be in pain, and if the disease isn't cured, will I die in pain?" In a study performed by the Institute of Medicine in 1997, 72 percent of cancer patients reported that pain was one of their primary fears after learning they had cancer, only slightly less than the number who feared dying. More than half of those surveyed believed dying of cancer meant dying in pain.

Many (but not all) persons who have cancer do have significant pain. The study mentioned above found that more than half of all cancer patients experienced moderate to severe pain at some time during their illnesses. In some ways, modern medicine is not nearly as aggressive at treating the pain as it is at treating the cancer itself. Good, effective treatment for pain is available; it's just not as widely available as it should be.

During the last decade or two, we've learned that there are many different causes of the pain experienced during cancer. Some of the causes respond well to the routine pain medicines every doctor prescribes regularly. Some causes don't respond to these medications very much, if at all. There are many less common treatments that can effectively relieve most of these other causes of pain. When needed, there are new, technically advanced treatments that can help control pain in almost every patient with cancer.

Unfortunately, many cancer patients in pain never get to try these treatments. This is no fault of the oncologists and other doctors who usually treat cancer pain. The simple fact is that these doctors spend several years of training after medical school learning everything they can about curing cancer. Usually, they also learn a lot about pain treatment, but it is never the focus of their training. In fact, 70 percent of oncologists (physicians specializing in cancer treatment) feel they do not know enough about treating pain. Even so, they are probably better trained in pain management than most physicians.

More than 85 percent of all physicians have never received any formal training in pain management during their internship or residency. They learned to prescribe for pain by writing the same orders the doctors a year ahead of them in training wrote. The average medical school curriculum provides two to three hours of instruction on pain medicines during the entire four years of instruction. Surveys of doctors in residency training (specialized training after medical school) have found that most of them don't even know how long the most commonly used pain drugs work after a single dose.

Taking Control of Your Pain

If you are in pain and know relief is available somewhere, then how should you go about getting it? One way, of course, is to have your oncologist refer you to a pain treatment center. There are one or two such centers in almost every medium to large city. For most cancer patients, a pain center is not absolutely necessary, however. Most oncologists and other cancer specialists already know a lot about treating pain. If a patient can help them understand what is causing his pain, they can probably treat it more effectively. They are also usually willing to try new medications and treatments when someone suggests them.

Many people simply tell their doctors, "It hurts, make it stop." Unfortunately, that's about as helpful as saying, "I have cancer, remove it." If the doctor doesn't know where the cancer is located, what type of cancer it is, and a lot of other things, she can't treat it well. We believe that the more you know about your pain, what is causing it, the effects it has on your body, and what can be done about it, the more likely you are to help your doctor stop the pain. In the case of pain, knowledge really is power: the power to suggest and receive the treatments that are most likely to help you.

That sounds simple, but it's not a simple task. Most people (including health care professionals) don't know very much about pain and know even less about how to stop pain. For that reason, we've included a *lot* of information in this book, including information about why pain occurs and the many different causes of pain. If you have cancer and are hurting right now, reading a book may not be your first choice as a way to get pain relief. You want to know what you can do today to make your pain better right now.

There are a few shortcuts you might take to speed things up, at least at first. If your pain medicine isn't working very well or is causing side effects, you can start with the pain medication chapters in Part II. That will give you some immediate information about alternative medications that you might suggest to your doctor. The other chapters in that part discuss some helpful therapies other than prescribed pain medications. The "alternative medicine" therapies discussed in chapter 9 describe techniques you can do at home and supplements you can start today, without a prescription.

Sooner or later, though, if you really want to understand why you hurt and find the best possible ways to stop hurting, you should read the other parts in this book. The first part discusses the many ways cancer can cause pain and the different types of pain sensations each mechanism causes. When you've read these chapters (and they are not hard to understand), you'll know more about pain and its causes than most doctors do. (No, we're not exaggerating. As mentioned above, few doctors have any real training in the causes or treatment of pain.)

Other chapters discuss the newest and most dramatic pain therapies. These treatments aren't miracles; they are just newer tools. But they may help people with certain painful conditions that can't be helped in any other way. Unless you understand the different types of pain, however, you probably won't be able to decide if these treatments are appropriate for you. If nothing else is effective, or if the cancer cannot be cured, there are chapters to help you decide if you want to try an experimental treatment or hospice care, and how to get them if you do.

Any medical information book, including this one, will have some limitations. It can't answer all your questions, or offer comfort as your loved one struggles with a serious disease. There are many organizations that can do just that, however, and the appendixes list dozens of support groups and research institutes, organized by topics. We urge you to contact an appropriate support group. It can provide new information that may have been released after this book was written, and some provide volunteers who can discuss your problems one-on-one, either in person or over the telephone.

PART I

What Causes Pain?

CHAPTER I

How the Body Senses Pain

by David van Alstine, M.D.

P ain is one of the most feared aspects of cancer. Many people believe that cancer always causes terrible pain that their doctors will not be able to treat effectively. It is true that many cancer patients do experience pain, and in some cases the pain is severe. However, cancer pain can almost always be treated and controlled effectively.

In order to understand the best ways to treat any particular pain, it's important to appreciate how the body senses pain. Many people have the mistaken idea that a pain message travels to the brain like a simple electric circuit; if you turn on the "pain" switch somewhere in the body, a "pain" light turns on in the brain. Actually, the pain-sensing system of the body is quite complex. Many factors modify the pain signals, either amplifying or reducing the amount of pain that is actually registered by the brain.

One way to think of the body's machinery for sensing and processing pain is to compare it to the telephone system. The phone system allows you to simply punch in a few numbers and talk to a friend in another state. Most of the time we don't care, or even think, about all the complicated things that must happen to call Miami from Dallas, just as we don't care how our body tells us that a cup of coffee is too hot to drink. We just want things to work correctly. When there is a problem with a phone call, however, it is important to understand how the system is organized. Otherwise, we would never know whether the problem is a broken phone, loose wiring in the house, a telephone pole knocked over by the wind, or a major failure of the telecommunications network.

The treatment of any problem, whether we are discussing telephones in the home or the pain-transmitting system in the body, depends a great deal on where the problem is located and what caused it. When your big toe is hurting, the doctor must determine if the problem is actually in the toe, in the nerves running down the leg, in the spine, or somewhere up in the brain. Just because you feel pain in your big toe does not always mean the actual problem is in the big toe.

In order to understand how the body's nerve network works and how it relates to cancer pain, it is useful to divide the pain system into three divisions: peripheral (out in the tissues) pain sensors, spinal cord processing of the pain message, and the brain's interpretation of the message. Once we have discussed how the nervous system sends a pain message (and it is much more complicated than most people think), we can discuss the ways that the nervous system modifies the pain signal.

In this chapter, we will also talk about the different types of pain. These have somewhat complex-sounding names, such as neuropathic (pronounced "new-row-path-ick") and visceral (pronounced "viss-err-all") pain, but understanding the different types of pain actually is not difficult. By knowing what bodily structure or structures cause a pain and what type of pain it is, a doctor can treat it more effectively. If you understand it yourself, it will not only be less frightening, but you can do a better job of explaining your pain to your doctor.

What Is the Difference Between Pain and Suffering?

The way the conscious brain senses nerve signals from the body is a lot like how a car radio picks up music. The various radio stations are always sending out a signal that carries the music, but you only hear something if you turn on your radio, adjust the volume, and tune in to one of the stations. The radio amplifies and modifies the radio waves into electrical signals that produce sound from the speakers. Because pain is so important a message, it can break through on any station, but the brain must be turned on and listening to get the message to the conscious mind. Pain consists not only of the signal the brain receives, but also the brain's own amplification of the signal and any mental or emotional reaction to the painful signal.

Before going further, it is important to discuss the differences between sensing pain out in the body, feeling pain in the brain, and experiencing suffering. Sensing pain in the body requires sensors to detect that something damaging is happening and nerves to transmit the pain signal to the brain. This part of pain perception is called nociception (pronounced "noe-sis-sep-tion"; "noci" refers to pain). Nociception includes not only sending the signal from an injured part of the body, but also any amplification or changes in the signal that occur as it travels through the spinal cord and brainstem.

The International Association for the Study of Pain (IASP), a group of health professionals and scientists with an interest in pain and its treatment, recognizes that there is more to pain than nociception. The group has worked for many years attempting to understand and define the other aspects of pain. They have recognized that although pain is something that all people have experienced to some degree, it is difficult to describe and define. In other words, it does not really mean anything to say that "pain hurts." According to the definitions of the IASP, pain is both a sensory and an emotional experience. The sensory experience is what we have just called nociception; the emotional experience, although definitely present, remains harder to define. Often, we refer to the emotional aspect of pain as suffering.

The actual sensations and effects of pain depend strongly on the individual who experiences it and the exact circumstances. We know that different people have different pain thresholds; some have a high tolerance to pain and some a low tolerance. For many years, it was thought that this difference in pain tolerance might be due to how strongly the pain signal was sent to the brain. However, we now know that when a group of people receive the same painful stimulation in a laboratory, there is very little variation in the signal that reaches each person's brain.

What does vary between individuals is the person's conscious and un-conscious reaction to the pain.

For example, if a man being tested for pain tolerance is being watched by a woman, he will tolerate more pain than if he is alone. Our culture promotes the idea that men need to be tough to be "real men." Some families strongly reward members with attention and pampering even for very small complaints, reinforcing the idea that tolerating even a small degree of pain is unnecessary. Other families give negative rein-forcement to members who complain of pain, teaching them that they should not complain. We learn these ideas about pain as children, and they stay with us when we are adults.

Each individual will also have a variation in his own pain tolerance at different times. During periods of high anxiety and stress, a person usu-ally has a lower tolerance to pain. This is especially true if there is a pe-riod of anticipation, knowing that a painful thing is going to happen. On the reverse side, a person may be so preoccupied with other aspects of a situation that pain is hardly felt. A soldier in battle trying to save his friends may suffer a severe injury without experiencing pain.

A person who has cancer usually is experiencing a lot of stress and anxiety that can change her tolerance to pain. In other words, she may experience more suffering from the same painful stimulation than she would at other times in her life. Even a minor pain might incapacitate such a person, who could ignore the same pain at other times. For ex-ample, a cancer patient who knows that the aching in his chest is caused by cancer spreading to a rib may have far more suffering than does a per-son who just had a major surgical procedure that cured his cancer.

Suffering and pain, although they often occur together, are separate issues. Grief, fear, anger, and depression can all cause suffering without causing pain. Childbirth may be very painful, but is usually not experi-enced as suffering. How much we suffer from pain will depend on things like our culture, our childhood experiences, our expectations, and the meaning we place on the pain. For this reason, a doctor needs to treat all patients individually and tailor a treatment plan for each person. At the same time, each patient may need to look at his own past and ex-pectations to see how these contribute to the suffering he experiences with his pain.

Peripheral Nociception
(The Sensation of Pain)

Every type of tissue in the body has special detectors that respond to stimulations such as heat, cold, stretch, pressure, position, pain, and many other things. The most important sensors for pain are actually the simplest; they are free nerve endings not attached to any specialized detectors. Any of the specialized detectors can also generate a pain message if they receive too much stimulation. For example, a temperature sensor usually sends "warm-cold" messages to the brain, but if things are too warm, it sends a pain message.

The free nerve endings, as the name implies, are just the end branches of a nerve fiber. When seen under a microscope, they appear quite similar to the branches of a tree. They generally send no messages to the brain until something damages the tissues. Like the smoke detector in a house, they are quiet as long as all is well. When activated, they fire off an electrical signal that rapidly travels up the nerve to warn the brain of a problem. On their way to the brain, these nerves connect to other nerves that may trigger certain reflexes to help us move away from the source of danger and damage.

Although the pain signal is electrical when it travels through a pain nerve, the stimulation that actually starts the signal at the free nerve ending is a chemical. A number of different chemicals, many of which can start a pain signal, are released when a tissue is damaged by injury, disease, or inflammation. Pain-stimulating chemicals include simple elements, such as potassium or hydrogen, and complex molecules, such as bradykinin, serotonin, histamine, and the prostaglandins.

In addition to causing the free nerve endings to send a pain message, some of these chemicals can "sensitize" the pain receptors, making them more likely to send another pain message if there is any further stimulation. If this increased sensitivity becomes severe, even sensations that are not normally painful, such as the brushing of fabric across the skin, can become intensely painful. The medical name for this hypersensitivity is allodynia (pronounced "al-oh-din-ee-ah"). Most people have experienced allodynia after becoming sunburned, when a simple pat on the shoulder can be pretty uncomfortable. The most severe cases of allodynia occur after certain types of nerve injury, such as the damage that may follow an episode of shingles.

The same chemical substances that stimulate a nerve ending to send a pain signal also cause other changes in the tissues, including changes in the smallest blood vessels (the capillaries). Among other things, the capillaries become dilated (swollen) and "leaky," bringing more blood to the area and allowing fluid to escape from the blood vessels into the tissues. This causes the inflammation (redness and swelling) that you notice after an injury. Swelling can help the body fight infection by allowing specialized white blood cells to travel into the tissues, but it can also contribute to pain and may cause other problems. The different chemicals have other effects, including attracting infection-fighting cells to the damaged area, increasing the ability of blood to clot, and, most importantly for our topic, causing pain.

Understanding the effects of these chemical substances has led to developing a number of medications that target pain and inflammation at the site of injury. For example, a large group of these chemical messengers are all produced from one "parent" chemical found in the walls of the cells of the body. When a cell is injured, this parent compound is released and modified to produce a whole family of chemicals called prostaglandins, thromboxanes, and leukotrienes.

All of the anti-inflammatory medications, such as aspirin and ibuprofen (Motrin and others), work in large part by stopping the creation of these chemical messengers. Aspirin (and the other anti-inflammatory medications) blocks the manufacture of these chemicals at the site of injury, reducing the sensitivity of the nerve endings. Tylenol (acetaminophen), on the other hand, has no action at the site of injury; it reduces pain by other mechanisms. This is the reason Tylenol works well for certain types of pain, while aspirin works best on other types.

Finally, the body does not just use one chemical signal to initiate the pain message and cause changes in the tissues. More than a dozen other chemical messengers are used to transfer the pain signal from one nerve to another—there are no direct electrical connections between nerves. It's not important to know all the chemical names of these substances or all the effects they cause. It is important to understand that a large number of

8

different chemical substances outside the nerves, as well as the electrical signals within the nerves, must work together to send a pain signal to the brain. In one way or another, almost every treatment for pain works by blocking the chemical and electrical transmission of these signals.

Transmitting Pain Signals to the Spinal Cord

As mentioned, the free nerve endings are not the only sensors in the body that can signal pain. All the other types of sensors (for temperature, movement, etc.) can create a pain message if they receive a strong enough stimulation. A little heat is not sensed as pain, but a lot of heat will be; a little pressure doesn't hurt, but a lot of pressure does. This is because the sensors, whether simple or sophisticated, send signals at a rate corresponding to the strength of the sensation. Each sensor is like a beating drum. The sensors are not capable of causing soft beats or loud beats; they can only change how fast they send signals. A little heat causes a temperature sensor to send a few slow signals. The temperature sensor sends the exact same signal rapidly and repeatedly when it is exposed to a lot of heat.

The brain and spinal cord are able to decipher this message by determining the type of sensor sending signals (heat, cold, pain, etc.), where the sensor is located, and how fast the signals are arriving. Brushing your finger over a candle flame sends a few heat signals to the brain, telling you it is hot and you should probably keep that finger moving. Resting the same finger in the flame causes a barrage of heat signals that the brain senses as severe pain. At times, this message is misinterpreted, such as when you place your hand in cold water, but immediately jerk it out again, thinking the water was too hot.

Each pain signal travels to the spinal cord along a single sensory nerve fiber. The cells that create the nerve fiber actually are located inside the bones of the spine in collections of neurons (nerve cells) called the dorsal root ganglion. Even though each cell is microscopically small, its "transmission line" is long enough to reach all the way out to whatever part of the body that the cell monitors.

These long nerve filaments are not all the same thickness, nor do they all have the same structure. The two most important types of pain-sensing fibers are called C-fibers and A-delta fibers. The A-delta fibers transmit pain signals to the brain very quickly because they are covered with a special insulation called myelin, which speeds up conduction. C-fibers lack this covering and transmit their signals more slowly.

How fast do these nerves conduct the signal? The slow C-fibers transmit their signal at about one and 1½ to 6 feet per second, while the A-delta fibers transmit at 40 to 90 feet per second. This difference is significant enough so that most people can clearly sense the different kinds of pain sensations carried by A-delta versus C-fibers. The fast-conducting A-delta message arrives first after injury. This pain typically feels sharper and "brighter." The C-fibers message comes a second or so later and tends to feel more dull and aching.

This has sometimes been termed first and second pain. After hitting your thumb with a hammer there is an immediate, sharp pain (the A-delta sensation), but this soon gives way to a deeper, throbbing, aching pain (the C-fiber sensation). If you don't remember the last time you hit your thumb with a hammer, trust us on this one.

Processing Pain Signals in the Spinal Cord

The system gets more complicated once the pain signal reaches the spinal cord, because a lot of different nerve cells all have to work together to get the pain message through to the brain. There is not just one nerve that carries pain information from your toe to your conscious brain, for example. The signal must be passed from the original sensory nerve to other nerves in the spinal cord.

Transmitting Signals from One Nerve Cell to Another

The place where two nerve cells interact with each other is called a synapse (pronounced "sin-aps"). At a synapse, the fiber from one nerve cell will come close to, but not quite touch, a fiber from another nerve. When a signal travels up the first nerve fiber to the synapse, the fiber releases a small burst of chemical messengers, called neurotransmitters.

The neurotransmitters drift across the small gap between the cells and bind to special receptors located on the second nerve fiber.

The chemical messenger does not always cause the next nerve to send a signal. Some synapses (called excitatory) make the second neuron more likely to send a signal, while others (called inhibitory) make the second neuron less likely to send a signal. Nerve fibers branch repeatedly, so each neuron may connect with as many as several hundred other neurons. When one neuron sends its signal, it may stimulate many other neurons, but each of those neurons may be receiving signals (either inhibitory or excitatory) from dozens of other neurons at the same time. When a secondary neuron receives enough excitatory signals, it sends a signal of its own.

All of this sounds incredibly complex, and it is, especially when one considers there are dozens of different neurotransmitters working at literally billions of nerve connections. However, the discovery of these neurotransmitters has greatly advanced many aspects of medicine. Many medications, including most pain medications, work by altering or mimicking neurotransmitters. Depression, for instance, can often be treated by medications that boost the amount of certain neurotransmitters in the brain. Higher levels of these molecules appear to "rebalance" the brain in a way that reduces the symptoms of depression, allowing people to resume more normal lives.

Neurotransmitters interact in ways we are only beginning to understand. Many neurotransmitters cause several different, and apparently unrelated, effects. For example, the same medications that are used to treat depression also help relieve certain types of chronic and cancer pain, even for people who do not have any symptoms of depression. It appears likely, therefore, that the same neurotransmitters that prevent depression are also capable of reducing pain.

Connecting to Other Nerves in the Spinal Cord

Once the pain message reaches the spinal cord, its signal is relayed to other nerve fibers that branch in several different directions. Some branches travel up the spinal cord to the brain, while others make additional connections within the spinal cord. For example, one branch may connect the sensory nerve to a spinal cord motor nerve (nerve cells that control a group of muscle fibers). This forms what is known as a reflex arc, which helps prevent more damage from happening to the body. If one steps on a hot ember from a campfire, the sudden surge of pain messages relay through the spinal cord, immediately signaling the leg muscles to contract, which jerks your foot off the burning coal. All of this happens as quickly as possible, without any conscious decision by the brain to minimize the damage to your foot.

Yet even this simple reflex can be controlled to some degree. Important relay and modifying centers in a portion of the spinal cord (called the dorsal horn) help process the pain messages. This area relays the signal up to the brain and connects to other nerves in the spinal cord, thus modifying their activities. If the coffee cup you pick up is too hot, your brain may override the reaction to drop it immediately and hold on long enough to set it back down without spilling. You've probably noticed yourself "stopping" a jerking reflex this way at some time.

There are also nerve fibers that travel down from the brain to this spinal processing area. These fibers can, among other things, actually dampen a pain message before it ever rises to the area of consciousness. This natural pain-killing system is one way that the body can reduce pain. The nerve fibers in this system use neurotransmitters that closely resemble opioid (morphinelike) medications. All of the opioid pain medications work, in part, because they stimulate areas in the brain and spinal cord that make up this natural pain-control system.

Transmitting Signals to the Brain

Other fibers in the spinal cord relay the pain signal up the spinal cord to the brain. The fibers from these pain relay cells are grouped into bundles, called tracts, as they travel up to the base of the brain. There are several different pain tracts, each traveling to a different part of the brain, where it then connects to other neurons. The major tracts are named for the part of the brain they connect to: the spinothalamic tract (connects to the thalamus), the spinoreticular tract (connects to the lower brainstem), and the spinomesencephalic tract (connects to the midbrain).

Cerebral Cortex

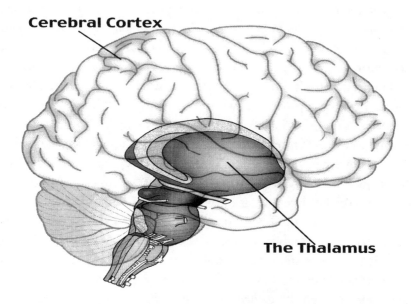

The Thalamus

Figure 1.1: The thalamus, an important relay center for transmitting pain messages, is located in the center of the brain, underneath the cerebral cortex (shown in light gray).

The next relay points are fairly complex, routing the pain signal from each tract to various parts of the brain. In essence, these connections (1) transmit the pain message to the conscious brain, (2) activate portions of the brain associated with motivation and emotional response, (3) stimulate parts of the unconscious brain that control things like blood pressure and sweating, and (4) interact with other cells that can modify the pain response.

The thalamus, in particular, is an important relay station for pain. It is located in the middle of the brain between the brainstem and the cerebral cortex (see Figure 1.1). Many sensory signals relating to position, sensation, motion, and pain travel through this area. From the thalamus, fibers transmit the pain message to the cerebral cortex (the outer part of the brain, with its wavy, noodlelike appearance). Damage to the thalamus can cause loss of sensation or the ability to move part of the body, but it can also cause unusual pain. Fortunately, this particular kind of brain damage is uncommon.

The cerebral cortex, which is far larger in humans than in nearly any other species, appears to be the conscious, "thinking" part of the brain. Some areas of the cortex have relatively specialized functions such as vision, hearing, and language, to name a few. Other large sections are less well understood. Although we do know in what area of the brain different sensations are processed (we know exactly which part of the brain feels sensations from the left index finger, for example), we do not know exactly how or where pain is sensed. There are large areas of the brain that do not seem to have a precise function except in broad terms like "planning" or "motivation." It seems likely that sensing pain involves activity in several different areas of the brain at the same time.

In addition to those sending signals to the thalamus, other spinal tracts carry pain signals to another area of the brain called the limbic system. The limbic system is not really part of the "thinking" brain, but rather is closely tied to our emotional state. It is not clear what purpose or advantage might be gained by transmitting pain signals to this emotional center of the brain. Perhaps, in less civilized times, it caused people to alter behavior so as to avoid pain or injury, or it motivated them to rest and recuperate after an injury.

Interestingly, the emotional response to pain differs greatly depending on the source of the pain. When an injury causes sudden damage, like a burn or a fracture, the emotional response is short-lived. It often includes irritability and sleepiness. This emotional response could obviously be helpful, since it could lead to rest and inactivity. When cancer or other chronic pain is involved, these connections deep in the emotional portion of the brain seem to result in more depression and anxiety. Obviously, emotional connections are less helpful in chronic pain, since this pain is usually constant in nature and does not change with rest. In chronic pain, the emotion connection only increases the suffering.

This is one reason that the most basic goal of treating cancer pain is to stop the pain signal before it gets to the brain, preventing the activation of these emotional centers. When this is not possible, the goal is to use medications and other tools to minimize not only the pain itself, but also the emotional consequences of the pain.

The Different Kinds of Pain

It is not intuitively obvious, but pain is not the same experience every time it occurs. A person can experience many different kinds of pain, partly because different parts of the body tend to cause or create different types of pain. Although severe stomach cramps and a toothache are both causes of pain, there are differences between those pains that are more than just the difference in location and intensity. Doctors classify pain into several broad categories to better understand what is causing pain and, more importantly from the patient's standpoint, how to treat it.

One way to separate the types of pain is by location, but from a treatment standpoint, this is not very useful. There is far more difference between toe pain and stomach pain than there is between toe pain and finger pain. It is more helpful to separate pain according to the kind of organ or tissue that the pain originates from, and the nerves involved in carrying the pain message. This kind of classification usually divides pain into five broad categories: somatic, visceral, neuropathic, central, and sympathetic types of pain. Each type has very different characteristics and may respond to different treatments, so each will be discussed separately.

In a complex disease, such as cancer, a person may suffer from more than one type of pain. It is important to understand each separate cause of a person's pain, since pain relief can only be achieved when each type is treated successfully. For example, a morphinelike medication should effectively relieve somatic pain from a bone, but will not help with certain other types of pain. If nothing is done about those other pains, the person still hurts, still can't sleep, and still has all the suffering that comes from chronic pain.

Somatic Pain

Somatic pain originates from the skin, muscles, tendons, ligaments, and bones. One can easily pinpoint the exact location of somatic pain, which is often sharp, stabbing, throbbing, or aching in nature. When you cut your finger with a knife, you know exactly where it hurts, even without looking, and exactly what the pain feels like. To some degree, these tissues can also cause referred pain (pain that is felt somewhere besides the actual point of damage), but when this does occur, the referred pain is typically located very close to the point of actual injury.

The parts of the body that cause somatic pain are particularly well monitored by the brain because they are so important to how we interact with our environment. You have to know where your feet are to walk without falling. In contrast, we don't really need to sense exactly where our spleen is located to perform everyday activities. The ability to describe exactly where the pain is coming from is handy when you need to take a splinter out of your finger. It also makes it fairly easy for your doctor to diagnose the cause of a somatic pain.

Although somatic pain can be severe, it tends to respond very well to a number of different medications and therapies. Most of the medicines created for pain relief work best to treat somatic pain. This includes medicines ranging from acetaminophen (Tylenol) and aspirin to codeine, Demerol, and morphine, among others. The effectiveness of any one of the medicines for a given cause of somatic pain depends on a number of factors. These include the severity and actual cause of the pain, the person's individual response to the medication, and probably even the individual's genetic makeup. (The use of these medicines is discussed more fully later in this book.)

Visceral Pain

Visceral pain is generated by the internal organs of the body such as the liver, intestines, or stomach. Visceral pain is often most severe when an organ is distended or swollen. In contrast to somatic pain, visceral pain tends to be poorly localized and more likely to generate referred sensations remote from the actual site of injury. The diffuse nature of this pain can make the diagnosis of its cause difficult and frustrating for both physicians and patients.

Luckily, some aspects of visceral pain can help identify its source. The hollow organs, like the intestines, typically generate an intermittent, cramping pain that may or may not have an underlying steady, dull pain. The solid organs, such as the spleen, usually cause a dull aching pain or pressure sensation. In addition, while the location of referred visceral pain cannot identify the structure causing the pain as exactly as somatic pain does, the pain does tend to follow certain general patterns. For example, an inflamed appendix usually first causes pain around the navel region. Later, when the wall of the abdomen overlying the appendix becomes irritated, the pain is felt in the right lower part of the abdomen where the appendix actually exists. Other common patterns of referred visceral pain are also known. Pain from the pancreas tends to radiate from the stomach straight through to the back, whereas irritation of the diaphragm (the main breathing muscle) is felt more in the shoulder. Unfortunately, these patterns are only helpful in general terms. When a person suffers a visceral pain, there are usually several different organs that might be the cause of that pain.

Cancer may cause visceral pain when a tumor invades an internal organ or presses on nearby organs. The treatment of visceral pain may involve medications, but routine pain medications are not as effective for visceral pain as they are for somatic pain. Fortunately, visceral pain associated with cancer often responds well to the destruction of specific nerve structures. (See chapter 10.)

It is relatively common for somatic pain and visceral pain to exist together. For example, a tumor from the colon or prostate that has metastasized (migrated) to a bone will cause both visceral pain from the original tumor and somatic pain from the metastasis.

Neuropathic Pain

Neuropathic pain occurs when the nerves themselves are damaged. This may happen when a tumor invades a nerve, when an episode of shingles destroys some of the nerve fibers, or when some structure presses on the nerve. Radiation and chemotherapy can sometimes cause neuropathic pain, although that condition is usually temporary.

Compared to other types of pain, neuropathic pain is typically more burning in nature, although it may also be perceived as aching. The area involved in neuropathic pain often has allodynia (hypersensitivity) even to a light touch. Some patients have lightning- or electrical shocklike spasms of pain that last for only a second or two, but which are dramatically more intense than the background pain. This has been termed lancinating pain and may require different treatments than the background pain.

Although it is sometimes convenient to compare nerves to the copper wiring in a house, the nervous system is made up of living tissue. As discussed earlier, there are several different types of nerve fibers. Damage to a nerve may completely destroy some fibers, but only injure others. The injured fibers may send abnormal signals that the brain perceives as a pain message, even though there is no "real" cause of pain in the tissues. Since some other fibers in the same nerve may be completely destroyed, it is not unusual for a patient to experience both numbness and pain in the same location.

There are two broad categories of neuropathic pain involving the peripheral nerves. Injury to a single nerve is often termed neuralgic pain. It can be caused by anything that damages the nerve, such as surgery, radiation, or invasion by a tumor. The other type of neuropathic pain can be caused by anything that mildly damages all the nerves in the body. Since the longest nerve fibers usually receive the most damage, the nerves to the feet and hands are usually most affected. This type of neuropathic pain, called peripheral neuropathy, causes a severe burning pain in both feet and sometimes both hands. Some forms of chemotherapy can cause peripheral neuropathy.

Neuropathic pain is not common in cancer patients, which is fortunate, because it is much more difficult to treat than either somatic or visceral pain. For example, morphine, which works well for many kinds of cancer pain, is sometimes completely ineffective for treating neuropathic pain. Fortunately, there are medicines that have been "borrowed" from other uses to treat neuropathic pain. These include drugs normally used to treat depression or seizures (see chapters 6 and 12). Additionally, nerve blocks and the injection of steroids (cortisone) near the affected nerves can dramatically improve some types of neuropathic pain. In more difficult cases, therapies such as nerve stimulation (see chapter 11) and certain nerve-destroying procedures (see chapter 10) may be attempted.

Central Pain

Central pain is similar to neuropathic pain in that it involves damage to nerve cells. In this condition, however, the damaged nerve cells creating the pain are located either in the brain or in the spinal cord. Central pain syndrome is rare. It usually occurs only after certain types of stroke or when brain tumors (including metastasis) involve certain areas of the brain. It often causes a widespread pain similar in nature to neuropathic pain, but very difficult for the patient to describe. It may also cause large areas of the body to become hypersensitive to pain.

Central pain can be extremely difficult to treat, although it sometimes responds to antiseizure medications and antidepressants (see chapter 6). Certain neurosurgical procedures may also be effective (see chapter 11).

Sympathetically Mediated Pain

This type of pain does not have anything to do with feeling sympathy for anyone; it simply refers to the sympathetic nervous system, part of the nervous system that controls involuntary or unconscious functions of the body. The involuntary nervous system is divided into two subclasses, the sympathetic and parasympathetic systems. These systems act in opposition to each other to maintain a balance between the various bodily functions. The sympathetic nervous system controls such functions as sweating, the actions of the intestines and internal organs, dilation and contractions of the pupils in the eye, and blood flow through various tissues.

The sympathetic nervous system is also capable of transmitting pain signals to the brain. In certain abnormal situations, the pain signals from the sympathetic nervous system become constant and severe, even though there is no obvious cause of pain. Physicians use a number of diagnostic terms when discussing sympathetic pain syndromes. By far the most commonly used term is reflex sympathetic dystrophy (RSD). Other terms used include causalgia (pronounced "caw-sall-gee-ah"), complex regional pain syndrome, and sympathetically mediated pain. Although there are slightly different definitions for these terms, in general they all refer to abnormal pain originating from the sympathetic nervous system.

The mechanism by which sympathetically mediated pain occurs is complex and not fully understood. The symptoms, which usually begin in a foot or hand, are often dramatic. Sympathetic pain has a severe, burning characteristic, usually without any aching or shocking sensations. The affected area is hypersensitive to even the lightest touch. Pink or bluish discoloration of the involved area may occur because of abnormal circulation, and abnormal sweating may be noticed in the affected area.

Like many pain syndromes, sympathetic pain is not directly caused by cancer but can result as a consequence of the cancer or cancer treatment. While uncommon, it is most likely to occur in persons who have either primary or metastatic cancer involving the extremities. It may begin after tumors invading the bones cause fractures of the arms or legs, after amputation of an extremity in an attempt to contain the spread of cancer, or without any specific inciting event.

Sympathetic pain responds to pain medications to some degree, but is usually treated more effectively with nerve blocks or destruction of the sympathetic nerves going to the affected area (see chapter 12). Since these nerves do not carry normal sensations, there is usually no long-term effect from destroying them. Unfortunately, the procedures are not always successful in relieving the pain.

Summary

In this chapter, we discussed how the body actually senses pain. We talked about the different types of pain and touched briefly on some pain treatments. In the next chapters, we will look at the specific ways that cancer and some cancer treatments actually cause pain.

CHAPTER 2

How Tumors Cause Pain

by David van Alstine, M.D.

T here are many ways that tumors can cause pain in the human body. Sometimes the pain is created directly by the tumor, such as when a tumor stretches or distorts normal tissues. At other times, the pain is caused indirectly by reactions to tumor-made chemicals, blockage of ducts from internal organs, bleeding into the tissues, collapse of bones, or other events. At times, the treatments used to fight the cancer can also lead to pain problems.

With all this talk about hurting, if you are newly diagnosed with cancer, it is important to realize that some tumors cause no pain at all, while others simply create a mild discomfort. Many people ignore unusual lumps or growths for too long; they assume it cannot be serious since it does not hurt. The cells that make up a cancer are from a person's own body, so they may not trigger a reaction from the immune system or from pain sensors. The body simply assumes that they are normal cells doing normal things.

One of the more futuristic ways to fight cancer cells involves creating special proteins called monoclonal antibodies that will stick to the cancer cells and suddenly make them visible to the body's own tumor-fighting cells. The goal of this type of treatment is to uncover the "stealth" cells that have turned cancerous and make them show up on the immune "radar" system.

Even when parts of the tumor have migrated through the blood stream or the lymphatic system and generated new metastatic growths, these may not cause pain. A look at the bone scan of a patient with metastatic cancer will often show several places that have been invaded, but are not hurting. For most cancer patients, there does eventually come a point, however, when the tumor causes pain. This may be even before the tumor is diagnosed, or not until late in the progression of the disease. Understanding how the cancer causes pain helps make sense of the treatments used to fight both the cancer and the pain.

Inflammation

As discussed in chapter 1, the initial sensation of pain and the transmission of the pain message to the brain are both chemical processes. At the edges of a tumor, cancer cells are invading normal tissue, damaging and destroying normal cells. These damaged cells release a few simple molecules, signaling surrounding cells and starting the inflammatory process. These molecules are modified by other cells to produce a large number of different compounds, resulting in a "cascade" of inflammatory chemicals. Some of these chemicals, like the prostaglandins discussed in the last chapter, are involved in causing pain.

It is important to understand several things about the inflammatory process as it relates to cancer and pain. The first is that these chemicals and reactions in the tissue are part of the normal mechanism the body uses to fight infection and to heal itself. Some of the molecules that are created attract infection-fighting cells to the area of damage; others make the blood more likely to clot, minimizing any bleeding into the tissues. Other cells attracted by these chemicals help clean up cellular debris, some may attack cancer cells, and still others create scar tissue to begin the repair process. Even the fact that inflammation causes pain is important, because pain warns us that something has gone wrong and motivates us to seek help.

There are times, however, when the whole cascade of inflammation and repair doesn't happen the way it should, such as when cancer cells escape being detected by the immune system and go on to badly injure the body. At other times, the response to injury or infection is more aggressive than needed for the situation. This happens, for instance, when a person is allergic to grass pollen or cat hair. The misery of a hayfever attack is caused by the body attacking something that is harmless and releasing a number of chemicals that trigger sneezing, watery eyes, and a runny nose.

When cancer first begins, the problem is less one of overreaction and more one of lack of detection. The tumor cells can be masters at hiding from our immune system since they arise from our own tissue, but at some point they begin to injure and start an inflammatory reaction. As the cancer cells grow and spread, they trigger pain through the inflammatory response. Although the reaction causes the same swelling and changes in blood clotting that an infection does, there is little evidence that this inflammation helps to fight the cancer.

Pain Originating from Different Tissues and Organs

In the last chapter, we discussed broad categories of pain, such as visceral and somatic pain. We considered the general way cancer causes inflammation and pain in any tissue it invades. It is also helpful to look at cancer pain according to the specific organs and tissues being affected.

There are several common ways that cancer causes pain when it infiltrates certain organs and disturbs normal function. Certain pains are best discussed by the organ affected, such as bone pain or nerve pain. In these cases, the pain is very similar, no matter what mechanism causes it. Other pains are best discussed by the actual mechanism causing the pain, such as compression, bleeding, lack of blood flow, and so on. In these cases, the mechanism determines the characteristics of the pain and how we should best treat it.

Bone Pain

Invasion of bone by cancer is, unfortunately, a common event. Although some types of tumor originate in the bone itself (like osteosarcoma; "osteo" meaning bone and "sarcoma" being a type of malignant tumor), more frequently the tumor originated somewhere else and then metastasized to the bone. Cancer of the breast, kidney, lung, and prostate are more likely to invade bones than are other types of cancer. The bones most commonly invaded are the vertebrae (spine), pelvis, and the long bones of the arms or legs.

Once cancer cells reach a bone, they begin to multiply, destroying healthy bone tissue as they grow. Sometimes the body fights back, forming new (although abnormal) bone at the site of a tumor, but bone destruction is the overwhelming rule. Bone invasion sometimes causes the most extreme pain experienced by cancer patients, while at other times it causes no pain at all. It is common for a person to complain of severe pain from an invaded rib, for example, but the same person may have several other ribs invaded by the same tumor that are completely painless. To understand the reason for this, we have to understand the anatomy of a bone.

The bones are made up of a dense mineral complex created by cells scattered within the mineral matrix. The mineral complex is the substance we usually think of as bone; the cells are few in number. The mineral matrix is continually remodeled by these cells, however, to help strengthen parts of the bone that are under stress. Most bones have a dense mineral matrix on the outside, with a central portion of lacy or spongy bone that contains spaces filled with fat and special blood cells. The spongy interior, called marrow, serves as the manufacturing site for new red blood cells, white blood cells, and platelets (which aid in blood clotting). The outer portion of bone is called the cortex. The dense cortex is the strong part of the bone that provides its main structure and support.

Overlying every bone is a tough, fibrous covering called the periosteum (pronounced "perry-oss-tee-um," "peri" meaning around and "osteo" referring to bone). The periosteum contains many nerve endings and is therefore the most sensitive portion of the bone. The cortex and marrow of the bone contain few nerve endings. When bone pain occurs, the periosteum is actually the source of most of the pain, with only a small contribution from nerves within the bone itself.

A tumor can spread to any bone in the body, but there is a tendency to spread into those bones closest to the tumor, called direct extension.

The direct extension of the tumor often occurs with lung or breast cancer that spreads to the ribs, or with cancers of the mouth and throat that invade the jawbone. However, direct extension can happen with nearly any type of tumor in any location. Direct extension usually begins on the outside of the bone and erodes inward.

Indirect extension of a tumor to bone happens when a few cancer cells migrate through the bloodstream or lymphatic system and lodge in a distant bone, a process called metastasis. Physicians and health care workers sometimes shorten this to "mets," as in the phrase "Mrs. Smith has bone mets." Metastasis can also occur to any bone, but it most commonly involves the vertebrae (bones of the spine), ribs, pelvis, or the long bones of the arms and legs. Metastases usually start in the central, blood-filled areas of the bone and erode outward as they grow.

When a tumor invades only the central part of the bone there is usually little pain, since there are few nerve endings located in that area. Whenever the periosteum becomes irritated, however, significant pain will occur. The irritation and stretching of this capsule causes a constant, deep aching pain that stress on the bone may worsen, such as when standing or moving. It is not surprising, then, that direct extension of the tumor to the bone, which irritates the periosteum immediately (since it begins on the outside of the bone), is usually painful as soon as it begins. Metastatic tumors, which usually begin in the center of the bone, are usually not painful until the tumor has grown enough to stretch the periosteum.

In addition to causing pain by irritating and inflaming the bone and periosteum, a tumor can cause pain by fracturing the bone. As cancer cells erode more and more of the mineral matrix, the bone continually weakens and eventually may fracture after no more stress than simply standing up. This kind of broken bone is termed a pathologic fracture because it does not involve enough injury to break a normal bone; it only occurred because of the pathology (disease process) of tumor invading the bone. For example, pathologic rib fractures may occur after simply coughing or sneezing, or a hip fracture may occur simply from getting out of a chair. There are numerous cases of a pathologic fracture being the first indication that cancer is even present.

Pathologic fractures are not only a major cause of direct bone pain but also can limit the patient from doing other activities that are important or pleasurable. The bone at the fracture site is extremely weakened by the tumor and will not heal easily or with normal strength. It is often necessary to surgically place internal support rods inside the bone, or to place metal plates and screws to bridge over the damaged area.

When cancer involves the bones of the spine, there can be serious problems with both pain and function. Since the spine must bear weight any time a person is sitting, standing, or moving, tumor-generated bone pain tends to be more constant and more disabling when it involves the spine. Additionally, if the tumor invades into the canals that house the spinal cord and major nerves, it can compress vital nervous tissues or even invade the nerves themselves. This can cause neuropathic pain (see chapter 1) in the nerves that are compressed and even stop the nerve from functioning, resulting in weakness or partial paralysis.

Like other bones, a vertebra (an individual bone of the spine) can fracture if the tumor destroys too much of its bone tissue. A pathologic fracture of a vertebra can sometimes cause catastrophic damage to the spinal cord and nerves and may require major surgery if the spine becomes unstable. Fortunately, most pathologic spine fractures do not cause significant nerve injury, nor do they require surgical repair. Such fractures do cause severe back pain, however.

Pain from the Nervous System

Another specific type of pain occurs when the nervous system becomes involved in the cancer. The nervous system is made up of the brain, the spinal cord, and the peripheral nerves, which progressively branch into smaller and smaller fibers to provide muscle control and receive sensation from the body. Cancer pain involving the nervous system happens when the nerves are invaded or compressed by a tumor, or when the brain or spinal cord begins to experience increasing pressure caused by the growth of a tumor.

Peripheral Nerve Irritation and Compression

The invasion of nerve tissue by cancer can generate severe and unique neuropathic pain (see chapter 1). Patients describe this as a deep aching or burning pain that is particularly distressing. It may include shooting electrical sensations (called lancinating pain). The reason this pain seems different from other types of pain is that the pain communication system itself begins to malfunction.

Damaged nerves are capable of generating their own signals, even when there is no real problem in the tissues they serve. These false signals are carried to the spinal cord and brain and may be interpreted by the conscious mind as bizarre and uncomfortable sensations. The pain of hitting the "funny bone" in your elbow is a good example of neuropathic pain. The shocks, tingling, and strange sensations running down to the fingers are very similar to what a patient with neuropathic pain experiences all the time.

It is interesting, though, that pressure and damage to nerve tissue is not always painful. Direct pressure on a nerve from scar tissue or a tumor may simply make the nerve stop functioning, causing paralysis or numbness but not pain. We still do not really understand what makes some types of nerve damage highly painful and others totally painless.

Unfortunately, nerve-generated pain can be difficult to treat with normal pain medications, even those as strong as morphine. Several studies suggest that nerve pain may only be one-third as sensitive to opioid (narcotic) drugs as other types of pain are. The reasons for this lack of response to opioid pain medications are poorly understood. The result, however, is that many patients are unable to obtain relief from neuropathic pain even with the strongest pain medications.

It is sometimes possible to treat this pain by either significantly increasing the opioid medication, though at the expense of more side effects, or by employing medicines typically used for other medical problems. These include steroids, antiseizure drugs, antidepressants, and a number of other compounds (see chapter 6). If it seems strange to think that a medicine for seizures might treat nerve pain, just remember that twitchy, malfunctioning nerve cells in the brain cause seizures, while twitchy, malfunctioning peripheral nerve cells cause peripheral nerve pain. The antiseizure medication stops either kind of nerve cell from malfunctioning as often.

Neuropathic pain usually does not occur until late in the course of cancer, although there is one notable exception. When lung cancer occurs near the top portion of the lung, it will often spread to the bundle of nerves that travels from the spinal cord in the neck, over the top of the lung, and under the shoulder to the arm. This nerve bundle, called the brachial plexus (pronounced "bray-key-all plecks-us"), is a large network of nerve fibers that come together to form the peripheral nerves of the arm. When a lung cancer invades this plexus, the affected person begins to have deep aching pain in the arm or shoulder that radiates down the arm to the hand. At times, the pain is accompanied by numbness and loss of muscle strength and coordination. This type of lung cancer is called a Pancoast tumor after the doctor who first described it. Unfortunately, a Pancoast tumor can be missed on simple X rays until it is far advanced because the collarbone, scapula (shoulder blade), and muscle of the shoulder hide this upper part of the lung.

Invasion of the Central Nervous System

Tumors that arise from or invade the brain or spine have quite different effects than tumors involving the peripheral nerves. The brain itself is insensitive to pain (it can even be operated on while a patient is entirely awake, as long as the scalp and the overlying tissues are anesthetized with local anesthetic). For this reason, when tumors arise within the brain, or more commonly metastasize to the brain, they do not directly cause pain. Patients with extensive tumor invasion of the brain often have absolutely no pain. They are far more likely to develop seizures or other neurologic problems.

In some cases, a tumor involving the brain does cause pain. When this occurs, the pain originates either from irritation of the lining around the brain (called the meninges, as in meningitis) or from increasing pressure within the skull. The skull is obviously not very expandable and is filled almost entirely by the brain. When there is bleeding within the skull, or when a cancer begins to grow and take up more and more space, then something else has to give way. Since the brain is suspended in a cushioning fluid, initially some of the fluid can be forced out of the skull to make room. At some point, however, the pressure within the skull begins to rise.

The first symptom of increased pressure is usually headache. The headaches associated with increased pressure inside the skull may, at first, vary in intensity or come and go throughout a day or a week. The headache is often worse in the morning, lessening in intensity during the day. Nausea and vomiting may also occur, again, usually worse early in the morning.

As the pressure increases, mental changes including drowsiness, sluggish thinking, and loss of coordination may become apparent. Double vision is another symptom of increased intracranial pressure, but is usually a late sign that occurs only after the pressure has become quite high. Any further increase in pressure causes the brain to malfunction and may eventually lead to severe problems with vision, coordination, and even breathing, as critical parts of the brain stop working correctly.

The treatment for this problem depends on where the tumor is located, the type of cancer causing the tumor, the extent of its spread within the brain, and the overall prognosis for the patient. It may make sense to operate on a single tumor that is located on the surface of the brain. Surgery is not an option when there are several tumors, or if the tumors are located in critical areas of the brain. Specialized radiation therapy may be the best option in such cases.

Other Ways Tumors Can Cause Pain

In addition to the direct mechanisms of tissue inflammation or irritation, bone invasion, and nerve compression sources of cancer pain, tumors can cause pain through more indirect actions. These effects include hemorrhage (bleeding), ischemia (lack of blood flow), obstruction of organs, and several other problems not caused by the tumor itself.

Bleeding (Hemorrhage)

Hemorrhage is the medical term for bleeding, implying loss of more than just a small amount of blood. A tumor can erode into a blood vessel wall, weakening it enough so that blood pressure inside causes the vessel to burst. Tumors also secrete substances that stimulate the formation of new blood vessels to supply the growing cancer. These blood vessels are not as strong as normal vessels, so they may spontaneously burst.

Whatever the exact cause of bleeding, the blood fills the local tissues, stretching and distorting them and causing a sudden, intense pain. Usually such bleeding occurs in a location where the surrounding tissues will contain the bleeding, and eventually the damaged blood vessel will contract and clot, stopping the process. The blood that has escaped into the tissue acts as an irritant, however, and can cause increased pain for several weeks.

Obstruction of Internal Organs

When a tumor is growing around or inside one of the tubular structures of the body, such as the intestines or a duct from an organ, it may become so large that it will obstruct the passageway. This obstructive process may have significant consequences depending on the location of the blockage.

When the problem happens in the digestive tract, the entire process of breaking down food and eliminating waste grinds to a halt. When the blockage occurs in the esophagus, it can cause food to "stick" in the throat when swallowing, which may eventually progress to the point that even swallowing liquids or saliva is impossible. Complete obstruction of the esophagus is uncommon, however, and usually can be treated surgically if it does occur. Even complete obstruction of the esophagus is not very painful, since the esophagus does not distend very much. (Distension is the major cause of visceral pain. See chapter 1.)

The stomach is rarely obstructed entirely because its internal size is so much larger than the esophagus above or the small intestine below. Although tumors of the small intestine are uncommon, other tumors (particularly those of the colon, pancreas, or ovary) can compress the small intestine, causing a small bowel obstruction. This type of obstruction can also result from scar tissue caused by prior abdominal surgery. When the small intestine becomes partially or completely blocked, it causes symptoms including nausea, vomiting, and severe, cramping pain involving the entire abdomen. This type of pain comes in waves and is referred to as "colicky" pain. Depending on how distended the intestine becomes, there may be an additional steady, underlying pain.

When the obstruction occurs in the colon, the symptoms are similar to a small bowel obstruction: nausea, vomiting, and colicky pain. Depending on the location of the narrowing, some patients may also have noted worsening constipation and very narrow stools for several weeks or months.

A complete bowel obstruction of either the small intestine or the colon is a surgically urgent condition. A patient will have a tube placed through her nose, down the esophagus, and into the stomach to help decompress the digestive tract. If the obstruction is complete, surgery will be needed to relieve it before permanent damage to the intestine results. Many cancer patients, however, suffer partial obstruction. That means the tumor is compressing the intestine enough to cause symptoms, but some food does pass through. The same symptoms are present, although they are usually less severe. Partial obstructions may be treated by nonsurgical means, although surgery may eventually become necessary.

Tumors can also block the various tubes and ducts that carry fluids throughout the body. Common sites of obstruction include the bile ducts (from the liver and pancreas into the intestines) and the ureters (from the kidneys to the bladder). Obstruction of ducts usually causes a cramping colicky pain that comes in waves. The pain is not as widespread as the pain of bowel obstruction and often refers to the organ involved. For example, ureter obstruction causes pain in the mid-back, while bile duct obstruction causes upper abdominal pain, often worse on the right side. Some types of tumor, notably cancer of the pancreas, are so likely to cause obstruction that even patients who cannot be cured have surgery to reroute the ducts and intestines in a way that helps prevent obstructions.

Tumors of the lung can cause obstruction of the bronchi (breathing tubes). Surprisingly, blockage of the breathing tubes is not painful and, in fact, may not even cause difficulties with breathing. It often leads to the development of pneumonia that will not go away, however, even when treated with potent antibiotics. This happens because the lungs are not able to clear mucus and dead cells from the area that is obstructed, and there is little air flowing to that region, a combination that provides excellent conditions for infection to begin. When pneumonia does develop, it may cause pain during deep breathing or coughing, but the actual tumor and obstruction is not usually the source of pain.

Obstruction of Blood Flow

Unlike the gradual blockage of an airway, obstruction of a blood vessel can cause a sudden, severe pain. Tumors can compress and distort small arteries within the body, eventually to the point that they block blood flow. When this happens, none of the tissue being fed by that artery receives enough oxygen and nutrients. Among other things, this causes the release of a series of chemicals, many of which trigger the pain receptors.

The eventual outcome of this type of obstruction depends on what part of the body the artery supplies and how complete the arterial obstruction is. When a complete, sudden obstruction of an artery occurs, some of the tissue it supplies will die, a process called infarction. Infarction of brain tissue causes a stroke (a cerebral infarction), while that of heart tissue causes a heart attack (a myocardial infarction). Obstruction of an artery caused by cancer, however, may happen slowly enough that the tissue can recruit other blood vessels to enlarge and supply nutrients. This new supply may be enough to keep the tissue from dying, but not enough to prevent the release of pain-causing chemicals.

Tumors can also compress and obstruct veins. This is especially common with tumors located in the lower abdomen and pelvis, which often block the veins that return blood from the legs. Some types of cancer cells can actually change the clotting tendency of blood, causing blood clots to form spontaneously in veins even when there is no tumor in that area. In such cases, it may become necessary to surgically insert a special filter to prevent clots from breaking off and going to the lungs (pulmonary embolus).

There are usually many more veins serving each part of the body than there are arteries, meaning that a number of veins can be obstructed without causing serious difficulty. When either many small veins or a few large and important veins from one area of the body become obstructed, however, it may cause serious problems. When enough veins are obstructed, all the tissue "downstream" (distant to the obstruction) begins to swell and becomes quite painful. Medications and elastic compression stockings may reduce the swelling, which usually reduces the pain.

Obstruction of the largest veins, the superior or inferior vena cava, can occur with certain tumors in the chest and abdomen. Vena cava obstruction can cause profound swelling and intense discomfort to almost half of the body. This problem is difficult to treat, and even the best treatments are rarely very successful. Fortunately, total obstruction of the large veins is not common.

Lymphedema

The lymphatic system is a specialized network of vessels (similar to veins) that reabsorb the small amounts of fluid that constantly leak out of the smallest blood vessels (capillaries). Like the veins, the lymphatic vessels combine to form larger vessels, eventually returning the fluid to the bloodstream. Without this system, there would be a slow but steady buildup of fluid in the tissues, causing swelling. Swelling from fluid buildup (called edema) has many causes, including allergic reactions, heart failure, venous obstruction, damaged tissue, and infection. Obstruction of the lymph system is a common cause of edema in cancer patients.

The lymphatic vessels are especially important in cancer because tumor cells can travel through the lymph system and establish new tumors in other locations. Within the lymphatic return channels are special collections of immune cells, the lymph nodes, that serve as screening centers for invading bacteria and other infectious organisms, as well as for rogue cancer cells. This is the reason that surgeons are especially concerned about removing and examining the lymph nodes when a patient undergoes a cancer operation. If the tumor spreads outside the original location and into the lymph nodes, the treatments required and even the chance of surviving the cancer may change.

If the cancer cells invade the lymph system, they may obstruct the fluid channels, causing severe swelling below the level of blockage. This type of swelling, called lymphedema, may also result from surgery if the lymph nodes are dissected. Lymphedema is more chronic and seems in some ways to be "thicker" than the swelling caused by obstruction of the veins. Many patients say the swelling from lymphedema is also more painful and interferes with movement more than other types of swelling. No matter what its cause, lymphedema can be difficult to treat. Radiation or chemotherapy to shrink the tumor may relieve the obstruction. Elastic stockings or gloves may reduce the amount of swelling. Sometimes specialized physical therapy with certain exercise programs can also help reduce the swelling and discomfort.

Shingles

Another way that cancer can cause pain is by causing shingles. Shingles are actually the reactivation of latent (inactive) chickenpox virus. Nearly all adults had chickenpox as children. An unusual feature of this virus is that it never leaves the body, even when the sores have cleared and full health returns. Instead, the virus lies in a dormant state in a portion of the nerves called the dorsal root ganglion, near the spinal cord.

The immune system usually keeps the virus suppressed, but the presence of cancer can weaken the immune system enough to allow the virus to multiply. Activated virus travels along the course of a single nerve root, reappearing on the skin as a painful rash called shingles. Unlike the original chickenpox infection, this secondary infection does not affect the entire body. It only shows up in the portion of skin receiving fibers from the involved nerve. Unfortunately, this reactivation is extremely painful. In severe cases, it can damage the nerve, resulting in months or even years of neuralgic pain (see chapter 1).

The medical name for shingles is *herpes zoster*. (This is different from genital herpes.) An episode of shingles that causes nerve injury and long-term pain is called postherpetic neuralgia. At present, there are a number of treatments that help reduce the pain of shingles and that also decrease the chance of developing postherpetic neuralgia. The treatments must be started soon after the shingles develops to be effective, however. If postherpetic neuralgia develops, it must be treated like other kinds of neuropathic pain.

Summary

As we saw in this chapter, there are many ways that cancer causes pain directly, ranging from irritation and inflammation of the tissue to obstruction of the intestinal tract and invasion and destruction of bones and nerves. Any patient may have different causes of pain at different times, or even at the same time. An understanding of the way cancer causes pain helps us to understand the medicines and treatments that are used to help relieve the pain. In the next chapter, we will look at how the treatments for cancer can, at times, be an additional cause of pain.

CHAPTER 3

Pain Associated with Surgery, Radiation, and Chemotherapy

by David van Alstine, M.D.

B efore exploring the way in which cancer treatments can cause pain, it must be clearly stated that this is not a case of the treatment being as bad as the disease. There is a common misconception that chemotherapy, radiation therapy, or surgery for cancer is a terrible ordeal to go through. In fact, although the process of chemotherapy can be very fatiguing and nausea is common, most of the side effects are either short-lived or easily treatable. Of course, surgery causes pain initially, but the body heals quickly from this. Radiation treatments tend to cause tiredness and skin irritation, but these conditions are usually mild and improve over time.

When the treatments themselves cause pain, it is generally only a temporary condition. In some (but not most) cases, the treatment may cause long-term pain, but even in these cases, it must be remembered that the primary purpose of the treatment was to cure a lethal disease. Even if the doctors prescribing it were absolutely certain the treatment would cause a long-term problem (and they were not), the treatment still would have been recommended.

In this chapter, we will discuss pain that arises from surgery, including pain that remains longer than expected, pain caused by radiation treatments, and pain resulting from certain chemotherapy agents. It appears discouraging that so many of the current approaches for treating cancer can be associated with pain, but the problem is less common than it was even a few years ago. As medical technology continues to improve, especially in early cancer detection, this problem will be minimized.

Pain Associated with Surgery

Most cancer patients will undergo some type of surgery, either in an attempt to remove the cancer or simply to get a piece of the tumor for biopsy so that the cancer can be accurately diagnosed. It is fairly obvious that surgery will cause some pain and discomfort, because there will always be some injury to normal tissues while the surgeon exposes and isolates the tumor.

Surgeons are trained extensively in the different approaches to various kinds of tumors. Their goal is to remove as much of the cancer as possible while causing the least amount of damage to other structures in the body. To some degree, it is the kind of tumor being treated that dictates what approach a surgeon must take, although the plan is adapted to each individual patient, sometimes even after the operation has begun. For example, areas of inflammation or infection can make a tumor appear to be larger or more aggressive on scans or X rays than it really is. Sometimes what seems to be one kind of tumor is found to be something different when the surgeon exposes it. In either case, the surgeon might find that a smaller operation than the one originally anticipated might be all that is required. On the other hand, cancer can be subtle and deceptive, sometimes requiring the surgeon to abandon a simpler procedure and perform a more extensive operation.

Unfortunately, there are times when a cancer has spread so much that surgery will not help cure the disease. Even in such cases, operations that relieve obstruction or reduce the accumulation of fluid may be necessary to help prolong life or prevent suffering. This type of surgery is referred to as palliative.

Incisional and Postoperative Pain

Much of the immediate pain after surgery comes from the direct trauma to the body caused by the scalpel and other cutting instruments. The various tubes needed to drain wounds, measure urine, or prevent the accumulation of fluid in the digestive tract all tend to be fairly uncomfortable right after surgery, but they are usually removed within a day or two. These types of pain that occur during the immediate postoperative period are called acute pain because they happen acutely (immediately) after the injury. Acute pain can always be effectively treated by a variety of medications. Usually an opioid (narcotic) type of medication will be used, since these are especially effective in stopping acute pain.

The pain of skin and soft tissue incisions usually resolves within a few days or weeks. However, some tissues may continue to cause pain long after the surgery. Muscle tissue is a common cause of prolonged pain after surgery. One reason is that injured areas in the muscle sometimes develop tight, small bands of spasm called trigger points. Because a tightly contracted muscle tends to cut off its own flow of blood supply, there is a tendency for these areas to deplete their energy reserves. Without proper blood flow, muscle tissue is even more prone to spasm, thus setting up a cycle of spasm and pain. For unknown reasons, this type of pain appears to become worse when patients do not sleep well. Unfortunately, since pain can be a major cause of sleeplessness, the whole process may become self-perpetuating.

Muscular pain is usually felt as a deep, dull ache, sometimes associated with a cramp or spasm of the muscles. The best therapies for this problem involve stretching the muscle through physical therapy and injecting the affected area with local anesthetic. Both types of treatment can stop the trigger point/spasm cycle and relieve the pain. A low dose of certain medicines that restore normal sleep patterns may also prove useful.

Another cause of prolonged pain after surgery is nerve injury. There are always small nerves that are cut during surgery, most of which will heal themselves within a few weeks or months after the operation. In a few cases, the nerve does not heal properly. Instead, a small ball of nerve

39

and scar tissue develops at the cut end. This is called a neuroma (pronounced "new-rome-ah"), and it causes pain both at rest and with movement. Neuroma pain usually originates from a small area near or in the scar. Pressing or moving the area creates a sudden increase in pain. Neuroma pain often is tingling or shooting in nature, so it feels quite different from either the pain from the original surgery or a trigger point in the muscle. Neuromas may respond to injection of the nerve with local anesthetic and cortisone, as well as to physical therapy.

Since a neuroma may not form for several weeks or even months after the surgery, patients may have a pain-free interval after surgery, followed by a new pain as the neuroma develops. Of course, most cancer patients fear this means the tumor has returned. The tingling, shocking characteristic of neuroma pain is quite different from the aching pain usually experienced from a tumor growing in the tissues, however.

Specific Problems After Surgery

A number of pain syndromes (syndrome means a group of related symptoms) are associated with specific surgical procedures. In many of these cases, it must be decided if the pain is coming from a syndrome related to the surgery or if some of the tumor remains and is causing the pain. Fortunately, there are usually specific signs that point in one direction or the other. In most cases, a CT or MRI scan of the area in question can show with relative certainty whether the tumor has returned.

Postmastectomy and Postthoracotomy Pain

About 5 percent of women who have a mastectomy (breast removal) for cancer will develop a condition called postmastectomy syndrome. The major symptoms are burning pain on the inside of the arm and armpit as well as on the chest wall. The skin in the area is often extremely sensitive to light touch, such as clothes rubbing across it. The pain is generally worse with motion, but is present to some degree at rest. Postmastectomy syndrome may occur soon after surgery, or may not begin for months after the surgery is over. Many women become particularly frustrated with this pain problem. Their breasts were not painful before the operation; but after surgery, pain significantly interferes with their lives.

Since movement is painful, affected patients tend to avoid moving the shoulder on the side of the operation. This can lead to permanent long-term loss of shoulder mobility (frozen shoulder) if the syndrome is not treated effectively. Medications and an aggressive course of physical therapy usually reduce the symptoms. At times, it may be necessary to inject areas in the muscles or under the ribs with local anesthetic and cortisone to help speed the recovery.

Similar conditions can occur following lung surgery through an incision between the ribs (a thoracotomy), surgery to remove a cancerous kidney, or neck dissection surgery. In all these cases, the symptoms are similar to postmastectomy syndrome. Of course, the location of pain varies according to the site of surgery. Whatever the location, however, the pain is always burning in character, worsened by movement, and associated with skin hypersensitivity. Depending on the operation involved, these syndromes are termed postthoracotomy pain syndrome (chest), postnephrectomy pain syndrome (kidney), and post–radical neck dissection pain syndrome, respectively.

What all these problems have in common appears to be damage to the small nerves and muscles around the incision. In the case of postmastectomy syndrome, a specific nerve that runs along the edge of the armpit, which is easily irritated or stretched during even the most careful surgery, is usually involved. Other nerves and the pectoral muscle (muscle under the breast) may also contribute to postmastectomy syndrome. Postthoracotomy and postnephrectomy syndromes often involve damage to the intercostal nerves (nerves running below the ribs). The muscles of the back or chest wall may also be involved in producing the pain of these syndromes.

These pain syndromes are difficult to tolerate, especially since routine pain medicines do not stop the pain very effectively. Fortunately, they do respond to certain treatments, and they slowly get better over a period of months. Treatments include medications that are effective against neuropathic pain (see chapters 1 and 6) as well as physical therapy to restore normal muscle function. Nerve blocks (see chapter 10) may provide dramatic relief, especially when combined with physical therapy.

Phantom Limb Pain

An unusual type of pain sometimes occurs after an arm or leg has been amputated because of the spread of a tumor (or for any other reason). After amputation, most patients experience what are called phantom limb sensations. These are sensations that feel as if the arm or leg is still present, even though it has obviously been removed. Phantom sensations are normal and usually go away in a few weeks.

A very few patients not only experience the sensation of an arm or leg still being present, but also feel that the missing limb hurts, sometimes severely. The limb may seem to be in an unusual position or twisted in a direction that would not be possible in life. This is called phantom limb pain. It seems to happen because the brain and spinal cord "expect" messages from all parts of the body. When a limb is surgically removed, there is difficulty in getting all the nerve cells to correctly interpret what has happened. We all have experienced such nerve confusion, such as when we put our hand in very cold water, but the water feels hot, or when pressure on the "funny bone" at the elbow makes our fingers tingle.

Phantom limb pain appears to involve not only the peripheral nerves but also their connections within the spinal cord. It is much more likely to occur if the amputated extremity was very painful before it was amputated. The condition can sometimes be treated with certain medications, or with physical therapy that stimulates the remaining part of the limb, though neither of these treatments is entirely successful. It may be necessary to perform neurostimulation (see chapter 11), which involves implanting an electronic device near the spinal cord to relieve phantom pain. The neurostimulator generates an electrical field that blocks the transmission of the pain message from the spinal cord to the brain.

Pain After Radiation Therapy

Compared to surgery, radiation therapy is often considered painless. Indeed, the vast majority of people who have radiation for cancer treatment never suffer any long-term pain. Of course, during the treatments there may be loss of hair within the radiation field and the skin may become mildly burned, similar to a sunburn. Some people also notice that any cuts or skin irritations in the area take longer to heal than they normally would. When radiation is given to the chest area, as for lung cancer or breast cancer, some people also develop irritation of the esophagus (food pipe). This is a bit like having a sunburn on the inside and can make swallowing uncomfortable.

Higher doses of radiation can cause scars to form inside the body, and this may result in long-term pain. For example, some patients who receive high-dose radiation to the mouth or throat develop damage to small nerves in the area, causing neuropathic pain. They also may develop scar tissue (fibrosis) on the inside of the mouth and throat that is painful when they chew or swallow. Similar conditions can occur after radiation to other parts of the body.

Radiation scar tissue presents a major problem when it involves a tubular structure, such as the intestines. All scars naturally shrink and become smaller over time. When scar tissue shrinks in a tubular structure, it causes the tube to narrow. This can result in obstruction and the types of pain associated with obstruction (see chapter 2). This problem was much more common in the past, but modern methods of adjusting the radiation dose and focusing the radiation beam have reduced the likelihood of this kind of problem.

High doses of radiation may also damage nerves directly or create internal scar tissue (fibrosis) that entraps nerves. Because nerve damage and scar tissue often do not develop for several months after the radiation treatment is completed, people who develop this complication often think that the cancer has returned. Radiation nerve damage can usually be treated with the same types of medication used for other forms of nerve pain. Internal scar tissue is very difficult to treat because whenever a scar is removed, the body simply replaces it with more scar tissue. For this reason, radiation fibrosis (scarring) is treated by methods that attempt to soften or loosen the scars rather than remove them.

The peripheral nerves and spinal cord can also be injured by radiation therapy, although, again, this is uncommon. Even when damage does occur, it is painful only 10 to 20 percent of the time. Radiation nerve damage is most likely to occur when the area receiving radiation contains a nerve plexus, a network of connected nerves that gives rise to the peripheral nerves traveling to the arm, leg, or another part of the body. One such plexus, the brachial (arm) plexus, is located at the top of the chest where it may receive radiation for a lung cancer. Another, the lumbosacral (low back) plexus, travels through the pelvis and may be irradiated when a pelvic tumor is treated.

Only a small number of patients who receive radiation to a plexus will develop problems. There are two common causes of radiation plexus damage. Damage to the nerve fibers themselves usually occurs a few months to a year after the radiation therapy has been completed. This type of problem can cause severe, burning pain, but it is usually temporary. Special testing, such as an MRI, may be required to make sure the pain is not caused by the return of the tumor.

The second cause of radiation plexus damage is actually caused by scar tissue that forms around the nerve bundle. The nerve fibers are not damaged by the radiation; they are compressed by the scar tissue. This may not occur until years after the radiation therapy has been completed. This type of damage is usually associated with weakness and loss of sensation in the affected area, but usually does not cause very much pain.

Like the nerves, the spinal cord can be injured by radiation. This is most common when the radiation is administered to the neck or to the mid-portion of the chest, but is still rare. Radiation damage to the spinal cord usually causes loss of sensation and weakness to the lower parts of the body. In a few cases, however, it causes a burning type of pain requiring specialized treatment.

A final type of radiation damage affects the bones. When radiation is given to an area of the body that contains a lot of bone, such as the jaw area or the pelvis, the radiation may damage or destroy the bone-forming cells. These cells normally repair and maintain the bone. If they are destroyed, that area of the bone fails to heal if it becomes damaged, is unable to fight infection, and becomes brittle and fragile. This is termed radiation osteonecrosis ("osteo" means bone and "necrosis" means dead). Osteonecrosis may be completely painless, but if a pathologic fracture develops (see chapter 2), it can be very painful. The pain of osteonecrosis usually responds to routine pain medications, however.

The chance of developing osteonecrosis depends somewhat on the location where the radiation was given, but mostly according to how much radiation was administered. This is one of the reasons that radiation therapy for cancer is only given by highly trained specialists. Carefully balancing the radiation dose hopefully provides enough radiation to kill the cancer cells, or to stop the pain when a cancer has spread out to the bones, but not so much that the bone cells are destroyed. The radiation is also focused on the tumor from several different angles, so that the normal tissue outside the cancer gets as little radiation as possible while the middle of the tumor receives a maximum dose.

Chemotherapy

The third major type of cancer treatment, besides surgery and radiation therapy, is chemotherapy. The success of chemotherapy depends on the fact that rapidly growing cells, such as cancer cells, will be more affected by certain medicines than will slowly growing cells. The goal of chemotherapy is to find just the right agent to kill the cancer cells without damaging the rest of the body. There are almost as many kinds of chemotherapy medications as there are kinds of cancer. Often several different drugs are used in combination to do the best job.

Even though our bodies seem to change quite slowly, the cells in some tissues are always being replaced rapidly, while cells in other tissues are only replaced over long periods of time. The cells lining the mouth and intestines, hair follicles, and the bone marrow cells that make new blood are all examples of tissues that must divide rapidly to function properly. One of the main difficulties in administering chemotherapy is getting rid of the rapidly dividing tumor cells without killing those normal tissues that also divide frequently.

Our ability to do this is only partially perfected. That is why patients undergoing chemotherapy often lose their hair for a while (it generally grows back) and have temporary decreases in blood cell counts. Until fairly recently, the ability to tolerate most types of chemotherapy was particularly limited by the ability of the bone marrow cells to tolerate the drugs. Too much chemotherapy caused anemia (lack of red blood cells to carry oxygen), problems with the blood clotting (because of a lack of platelets), and trouble fighting infection (because of a lack of white blood cells). Advances in treatment now allow the transfusion of red blood cells and platelets when necessary. Doctors can even administer artificial hormones to stimulate the patient's own blood cell production. This allows doctors to give higher doses of chemotherapy, resulting in more effective treatment of the cancer. Unfortunately, higher doses of chemotherapy may also make some painful complications more likely to develop.

As with radiation therapy, chemotherapy is a cornerstone of cancer treatment. It is a life-saving treatment for a lethal disease, so potential complications (other than those that might themselves be lethal) must be tolerated and treated as necessary. Avoiding chemotherapy because of the potential complications should not even be considered.

Some types of chemotherapy can cause pain when they are given and for a few days afterward. Corticosteroids (also called steroids or cortisone) that are given along with some types of chemotherapy may result in pain when they are stopped. Both these types of pain are temporary, however, and usually respond well to routine pain medications.

There are some long-lasting painful conditions associated with chemotherapy. Certain chemotherapy drugs can cause widespread damage to nerves, called peripheral neuropathy. Peripheral neuropathy caused by chemotherapy usually results in a burning pain in the hands or feet. Stimulation may worsen the pain, such as from clothes rubbing against the skin or exposure to heat or cold. There may also be other sensations that show the nerves are not working properly, similar to the "pins and needles" sensation we have all experienced after crossing our legs too long. Unlike other forms of nerve damage associated with cancer, peripheral neuropathy usually affects both sides of the body equally.

The likelihood of peripheral neuropathy varies depending on the type of chemotherapy used. Many chemotherapy medications rarely, if ever, cause the problem. With one class of chemotherapy drugs called the vinca alkyloids, nearly 100 percent of patients will have some burning discomfort in the hands and feet while they are receiving the medication. Other chemotherapy drugs that are frequently associated with peripheral neuropathy are:

- Vincristine
- Vinblastine
- Cisplatin
- Paclitaxel
- Procarbazine
- Misonidazole
- Hexamethylmelamine

None of these drugs causes neuropathy in every case, but if your specific cancer requires treatment with one of the drugs on the list, you may develop the problem. Again, this does not mean you should not use this type of chemotherapy. The problem of peripheral neuropathy can be treated if it does occur, and it is certainly less important than curing the cancer.

Some of the other chemotherapy medications sometimes cause specific pains, usually for reasons we do not understand. For example, vincristine can cause pain in the jaw. Interferon often causes the bones and muscles to ache as they might when you have the flu. Transretinoic acid may cause widespread, aching pain in the bones, while L-asparaginase can cause headaches. All these symptoms are temporary and can be effectively treated by routine pain medications when they do occur.

In certain cases, chemotherapy is given directly into one part of the body, rather than simply injected into a vein. Certain types of direct chemotherapy have their own associated pains. For example, when chemotherapy is given directly into the liver or the abdomen, about 25 to 50 percent of people will experience significant abdominal pain. This is temporary, but may require the use of strong opioid (narcotic) pain medicines for several hours or a day after the therapy. When methotrexate is given directly into the spinal fluid (as is done to treat certain brain tumors), it may cause headaches. These headaches result from irritation to the meninges (the tissue lining the fluid-filled space around the brain). They can be treated effectively with opioids or anti-inflammatory medications and do not cause long-term pain.

Corticosteroids (Cortisone)

Corticosteroid (cortisonelike) drugs are used frequently in the treatment of cancer. These are not the kinds of steroids that bodybuilders use to gain muscle; they are anti-inflammatory steroids. These medications can help chemotherapy kill certain types of tumor cells. They are also used to diminish the swelling around a tumor that may occur when other treatments kill cancer cells. Swelling around the tumor is especially important in cases of brain cancer, when swelling could put pressure on the brain, causing life-threatening problems. Corticosteroid medications, including prednisone, methylprednisolone, and dexamethasone, are the most effective weapons doctors have against such swelling.

Controlling swelling around some tumors is often an important method of reducing the pain from certain types of cancer. However, patients who have been on corticosteroids (sometimes only for a few weeks) may develop severe pain in their joints when the medication is stopped. This has been termed steroid pseudorheumatism, meaning that it seems similar to the joint pain experienced by patients with rheumatoid arthritis. The treatment for this condition is to put the patient back on steroids and then slowly taper off the dose over several weeks.

High doses of corticosteroids may occasionally cause pain in the groin area in a few people. There is no effective treatment for this pain, other than symptom relief with opioid pain medications. Finally, a small number of patients who require steroids for a long period of time (months or years) develop a problem with the blood supply to the hip or shoulder joints. This leads to the death of a section of bone, which can cause pain and increase the chance of fracture. The therapy for this condition (called avascular necrosis) may involve surgery to remove the damaged bone and replacement with an artificial joint or metal hardware.

Summary

Some of the treatments for cancer, including surgery, radiation, and chemotherapy, can occasionally cause pain. A basic principle of medicine is that the amount of risk taken in treating a disease depends on the risk of not treating the disease, and on how successful the treatment is likely to be. With cancer, it is almost certain that without treatment the tumor will spread and eventually be fatal. Even if there is a significant chance that the treatments will cause temporary or sometimes lasting pain, the benefits far outweigh the risk. When cancer treatments do cause pain, the pain is nearly always treatable, whereas an untreated cancer is nearly always fatal. For this reason, no patient should worry about the long-term effects of cancer treatment. Any painful problems can be treated as they arise.

CHAPTER 4

Other Factors That Worsen Pain and Suffering

by Roger S. Cicala, M.D.

Psychological Factors — It's Not in Your Head

For some people, the very existence of this chapter will be irritating. As soon as the words *psychological factors* are mentioned in the same discussion with pain, they immediately respond "It's not in my head." Of course, it's not. However, it's just as silly to say that emotional and other factors do not have any influence on the pain a cancer patient experiences. Literally thousands of studies say otherwise.

For example, every patient with significant pain, whether from cancer or other causes, knows several things that tend to modify his pain. Pain often gets worse following stressful situations, such as a fight with a loved one. Sudden changes in the weather may make the pain worse. Many people find that pain is different at different times of the day. Some people wake up with more severe pain, while others find that pain is worse in the evening when they are tired.

More importantly, when pain is defined in its broadest terms as "any sensation that the patient feels is uncomfortable," we must reconsider exactly what pain is. Being tired from a sleepless night is uncomfortable. Being depressed and hopeless is uncomfortable. Being tense and anxious is uncomfortable.

As a group of doctors who deal only in treating pain, we all believe that it is our job to address all the uncomfortable sensations a patient experiences. For this reason, we think it is very important to specifically treat depression, anxiety, sleeplessness, or any other sensation that is uncomfortable to our patients. These sensations are real when they occur. They contribute to pain, suffering, and distress. No one cares why they are there; they are simply problems that should be addressed.

However, it is important to treat each specific type of symptom with an appropriate medication or therapy, simply because that is the most effective way to feel better. An extra pain pill at night, for example, often helps someone sleep better when she is restless. To be perfectly honest, most people who take pain medication regularly have done just that— taken an extra pain pill so they could sleep a little better. They probably did have pain that night and decided perhaps the pain was why they could not sleep.

The truth is, though, that taking a sleeping pill probably would have been more effective. Although taking an extra pain pill one night is not a problem, taking an extra one every night may lead you and the doctor to think the pain medicine has not been working well. That may lead to a change in medication that is not necessary, and the new medicine may cause new side effects. In the same way, an extra pain pill may help reduce anxiety. It may even help relieve depression for a short time, although it often makes the depression worse, eventually.

The simple fact is that American culture has developed a myth that it is not acceptable to be depressed or anxious, particularly if you are an adult male. Although we probably know better, many of us get caught up in this idea that feeling depressed or anxious somehow means we are mentally or emotionally weak. However, in American culture it is quite acceptable to be in physical pain. Unfortunately (at least from a pain doctor's point of view), by the time many of us become adults we have almost lost the ability to know if we are depressed, anxious, or anything else. We simply know we are uncomfortable. If we are uncomfortable and also have physical pain, we tend to attribute all our emotional discomfort to the physical pain.

Factors other than physical pain contribute to almost every cancer patient's discomfort, and these factors can actually worsen the physical pain. Most people who suffer chronic pain have more severe pain when they do not sleep well, when they become anxious, or when they are badly depressed. Treating each of these symptoms with the right medication or therapy not only relieves that symptom, it also helps the pain medication relieve the pain more effectively. This sounds very simple, but actually it can be quite complex.

Very often, it is quite difficult for a person to know exactly why he feels uncomfortable. However, if you want to feel as good as you possibly can, it is important to carefully consider, with an open mind, what other symptoms could be contributing to your discomfort. You will have to mention them to your doctor, too. She cannot provide effective treatment unless you let her know exactly how you feel.

Depression

It is amazing that some cancer patients do not suffer depression. Being told he has cancer is one of the most catastrophic events a person can face. Fear, sadness, and grief occur in every person who hears this news. Most people experience violent mood swings afterward, with episodes of denial, despair, fear, irritability, and depression. Almost everyone who is told that she has cancer experiences insomnia for weeks or even months.

Before the cancer patient has had any real chance to regain his emotional balance, his life will be disrupted by surgery, chemotherapy, diagnostic tests, and the constant waiting for results. Few people receive universally good news after every treatment or test, and every bit of bad news creates even more emotional turmoil. First things look better, then they do not. Sometimes the doctors are not sure what this or that test means.

Added to this are the physical symptoms caused by the disease and its treatment. Hair loss or disfigurement from surgery and chemotherapy may occur. Nausea and vomiting can become a constant part of life. Pain may be severe at times. Cancer and many of the treatments all cause fatigue. And always, there is anxiety about what might come next. The stress and anxiety add even more fatigue and exhaustion.

So it truly is amazing that some people bounce back emotionally within a few weeks or months. Many others, however, find that they become increasingly hopeless and depressed. Between 20 and 25 percent of all cancer patients meet the psychiatric criteria for major depressive syndrome during at least part of their illness. Persons with significant pain, advanced cancer, and certain types of cancer are even more likely to suffer depression than other cancer patients.

Many people immediately respond, "Well, who wouldn't be depressed?" Of course, almost every person would be depressed in these circumstances. The point is not why a person is depressed or if she should be depressed. The point is that the depression itself makes things worse. It is not necessary to suffer with the symptoms of depression, even if there is every reason to be depressed.

No one chooses to suffer through the chain of events that lead to major depression. However, when this depression does occur, many people avoid or ignore treatment. As a psychiatrist colleague once said, "I've never met a patient who volunteered to develop depression, but I've met a lot who volunteered to keep it."

Many people assume that the medications and therapies used to treat depression only work for those people who have become depressed for no apparent reason. They do not realize that treatment for depression can be very effective even when the depression is caused by a person's situation and circumstances. In fact, some studies show that cancer patients respond to antidepressant medications more readily than most other people with depression do.

In case you are wondering, being depressed does not mean you have to see a psychiatrist. Any doctor can prescribe antidepressants. Most oncologists and pain doctors do so regularly. Of course, antidepressant medications cannot make you feel happy and wonderful all the time. They can, however, lift spirits, lessen sadness, and dramatically help the other symptoms of depression, such as sleeplessness, constant worrying, and irritability.

Few physicians will ask about depression symptoms unless the patient volunteers them, though. Most oncologists, for instance, focus on treating the disease itself. They often assume the patient will mention any other symptoms that are bothering him. However, many patients find it difficult to say they are depressed, or they assume (often incorrectly) that their doctors are aware of such depression. And so, the subject may never come up for discussion.

If the subject is not discussed, then treatment is not started. One recent study found that only 3 percent of cancer patients ever received antidepressants. Another study found that only 20 percent of cancer patients considered to be severely depressed ever received treatment for their depression. Those cancer patients that did receive antidepressant treatment, however, not only reported that they felt much better, but they gained more weight and had less pain than those not taking antidepressants.

What Does Depression Have to Do with Pain?

Considering the focus of this book, it is especially important to realize that pain and depression are closely related. Everyone can understand that having pain that is not treated adequately can worsen depression. It's important to realize, however, that having depression that is not adequately treated is just as likely to make the pain worse. This happens for several reasons. For simplicity's sake, we can group them into conscious, unconscious, medical, and chemical reasons.

Conscious Reasons for Depression

The conscious reasons are the easiest to understand and are the ones that most depressed people will deny, even to themselves. When a person is severely depressed, he does not want to do anything. Some days, just getting out of bed takes more effort and energy than he has. Yet, it's extremely rare for anyone to say, "I'm just too depressed to get up today." Even if he did, family members would probably nag him into getting up anyway. However, it is acceptable to say, "I just hurt too bad to get up today," and in this case family members are likely to leave him alone. Many of us learned this as children. "Mom, I really don't feel like going to school today" did not work. "Mom, I really feel sick" worked at least some of the time.

Unconscious Reasons for Depression

A similar effect can be caused by the unconscious mind. A severely depressed person knows she does not feel like getting out of bed, but is unsure why she feels so bad. The explanation must be that she's sick. If, in order to detect what might be wrong, she lay in bed concentrating on her symptoms, they would seem worse. After a few days of lying in bed, physical changes occur that add to the pain: the joints stiffen, muscles begin to ache, and bowel and bladder function is impaired.

Medical Reasons for Depression

Another unconscious process can lead to interactions between depression and the opioid (narcotic) pain medications. On a short-term basis, many of the opioids make people feel a bit euphoric (happy). Obviously, this might make a depressed person feel better. The natural conclusion is: "Since I feel better when I take a pain pill, I must be depressed because of the pain." The only real problem is that the euphoric effect wears off after a while, and a higher dose of pain medicine is needed to get it back. Pretty soon, the person is taking a lot more pain medicine than he might need to stop the pain. When high doses of opioids are taken for a long enough time (a week or two may be enough), the euphoric effect may actually reverse, and the pain medicine makes the depression worse.

In some cases, the depression is so severe that the affected person can hardly stand to be awake; she just feels miserable. Since another side effect of some pain medicines is sedation, she may start taking pain medicine or tranquilizers to make herself sleep. In a way, this makes sense— she uses the pain medicine to stop feeling the emotional pain. The sedation side effect stops working even more quickly than the euphoric effect, however.

Chemical Reasons for Depression

The chemical relationship between pain and depression is perhaps the most important reason depression should be treated in cancer patients. Most people are aware that parts of the brain can suppress pain signals (see chapter 1 if you are not). In fact, these areas of the brain are active most of the time, suppressing minor aches and twinges that we do not really need to know about. The cells in the pain-suppressing areas of the brain release certain chemical neurotransmitters to suppress pain signals. Many studies have shown that the levels of these chemicals are much lower in people with significant depression than in other persons. It has also been shown that depressed persons have an increased sensitivity to pain. When the depression is treated, the chemical levels return to normal, and the increased sensitivity to pain is reduced.

For all these reasons, it is very important to treat depression when it becomes severe, no matter how "appropriate" the depression may be. Obviously, there will be times when every cancer patient will feel depressed for a while. When the depression worsens, the person's quality of life for a significant amount of time, no matter how many reasons there are for the person to be depressed, it should be treated. This is especially important if the person suffers both pain and depression, since pain treatment will be much more effective if the depression is also treated.

What Is a "Normal" Degree of Depression for Cancer Patients?

Almost every cancer patient will suffer some degree of depression, at least for a while. When they first learn that they have cancer, most people experience feelings of disbelief, despair, or denial that generally last a week or two. After this, they may continue to experience insomnia, anxiety, loss of appetite, irritability, obsessive thoughts, and fears about the future. This often results in difficulty concentrating and remembering things, severe enough to interfere with the ability to perform everyday tasks. Even driving can be dangerous, because it is so difficult to concentrate. Most people return to a near normal mental state within a few weeks. However, many people continue to experience brief periods when some of these feelings return, especially during times of anxiety or stress.

About half of all cancer patients will have enough difficulty during this "normal" adjustment period that they may need a mild tranquilizer or at least a sleeping pill. It is important to use just enough of this medication to lessen the anxiety. A few people want to take so much that they sleep all the time. Although being unconscious does allow them to avoid the awful feelings they may have when they are awake, eventually they will still have to deal with those feelings. In other words, if you don't deal with it now, you'll just have to deal with it later. The purpose of a tranquilizer is to allow you to deal with the feelings without suffering severe anxiety.

A few cancer patients never seem to pass through this difficult time, however. Some remain very anxious and depressed for months. Others may have almost total denial of having cancer at first. Months later they may begin to suffer anxiety and depression when the reality of their condition sinks in. In either case, the depression and anxiety, while understandable, can interfere with the ability to fight disease. And this makes the patient, and his loved ones, miserable.

It's important for family members to understand that severe depression does not always appear as sadness. It often involves lack of energy, the inability to enjoy anything (called anhedonia), irritability, and sometimes anger or hopelessness. About 5 percent of otherwise healthy people suffer this degree of depression at some point during their lives. Most studies show that between 35 and 50 percent of cancer patients become this depressed, at least for a period of time.

Listed below are factors that can cause severe depression in a cancer patient.

Cancer-Related Factors
- Untreated pain
- Marked physical limitations
- Tumors of the lung, pancreas, colon, breast, or brain
- Malnutrition
- Hormone-secreting tumors
- Medications and treatment
- Steroids
- Opioids (particularly in high doses for a long time)
- Certain chemotherapies (vincristine, vinblastine, procarbazine, and others)
- Interferon or interleukin therapy
- Antiviral medications
- Brain radiation or intrathecal (in the spinal fluid) chemotherapy

Other Factors

- Past history of depression
- Past history of anxiety disorder
- Alcoholism or substance abuse
- Additional life stresses
- Absence of family or social support
- Family history of cancer
- Anemia
- Age older than sixty

Hospitalized or bedridden patients are more than twice as likely as other cancer patients to have severe depression. Cancer patients with significant pain that is not treated effectively, those who have had major surgical procedures, and those with breast or lung cancer are all more likely to become depressed. Older patients are more likely to suffer depression than are younger patients with the same type of cancer. In older patients, however, depression often causes symptoms of confusion and anxiety.

When Is Depression Severe Enough to Need Treatment?

Anhedonia, the state in which nothing seems pleasurable, is probably the most common warning sign of severe depression in cancer patients. When things that have always been pleasurable, such as a visit from grandchildren or watching a favorite TV show, just do not seem worth the effort, severe depression may be beginning. Other clear warning signs of depression include irritability (or even angry outbursts), increased anxiety, and hopelessness.

Some of the symptoms normally considered signs of depression, such as loss of appetite, difficulty sleeping at night, low energy levels, diminished sexual drive, and increased fatigue, are common in cancer patients whether they are depressed or not. However, when these symptoms are more severe than would be expected, or when they worsen even though the person's physical condition improves, depression may be the cause.

In many cases, it is obvious that some depression is present, but no one (including the patient) is certain if the depression is significant enough to require treatment. In such situations, a trial of antidepressant medication lasting two or three weeks is usually worthwhile. The newer antidepressants have few side effects and may help dramatically. If they are not helpful, they can always be stopped.

Treatment of Depression in Cancer Patients

When depression becomes severe enough to be treated, any of several different therapies can be helpful. The two general approaches to treating depression are counseling (sometimes called psychosocial therapy) and medication. The most effective treatment for severe depression usually combines both.

Counseling. Counseling can take many different forms, which can be individualized to best help with the problems and concerns of each patient. Most cancer patients do not require individual psychotherapy to treat their depression, but many do find that a lay therapist, minister, or support group experienced in working with cancer patients is a wonderful help. Most cancer centers offer individual and group counseling for patients, family members of cancer patients, and patients and families together.

Many cancer patients find that in some ways they cannot relate or speak freely to the people they love. They do not want to talk about their worries or sadness to family members for fear of making them worried or depressed. Talking to other cancer patients in a support group or to therapists who work with cancer patients regularly can provide a wonderful outlet. Cancer education groups can do wonders to relieve the fears and anxieties about "what will happen next."

Family members can also benefit from counseling. Most cancer centers sponsor group sessions with family members of other cancer patients and cancer survivors. The sessions might include education about the disease and treatments, teaching coping skills that help combat feelings of helplessness, and simple ways to deal with the stress of cancer treatment. The groups are often associated with social workers who can help with real-world problems, such as finances, transportation, and getting help at home.

If you are having any problems locating the kind of support group you are interested in, Appendix D lists dozens of national organizations that can put you in touch with a local support group.

Medications. (*Note:* This part discusses antidepressant medications in some detail. Many of the same medications are also mentioned in chapter 6, because they have significant pain-relieving qualities in addition to their antidepressant effects. In order to avoid confusion, the emphasis of this chapter is on the antidepressant effects of these medications, while chapter 6 focuses on using antidepressants to treat pain. There are some differences in the choices and recommendations of the various antidepressant medications, depending on the primary purpose for which they are being used.)

Antidepressant medication is the most effective treatment for severe depression. Some people are very resistant to the idea of taking antidepressants because they feel the medication is a crutch, or that they should be able to cope on their own. From a logical point of view, this makes just as much sense as thinking, "I should be able to walk on this broken leg without a crutch." Crutches serve an important, although temporary, purpose by allowing the body to heal. For most cancer patients, antidepressant medication is something they need to take for only a few months, not for years.

Other people remember that when Aunt Mary took antidepressants ten years ago, she was sleepy all the time or had some type of reaction to the medication. There are literally dozens of antidepressants marketed today that were not available as recently as 1990. More than half a dozen new antidepressants have been introduced in the last three years alone. Compared to what was available even a decade ago, today's antidepressants are more effective, work more quickly, and have far fewer side effects.

As mentioned earlier, severe depression means that certain chemicals in the brain are not present in their normal amounts. These low chemical levels are the reason that depression interferes with several bodily functions such as sleeping, eating, and tolerating pain. Antidepressants can restore these chemicals to more normal levels, relieving most of these other symptoms in addition to treating the depression. In fact, because antidepressants can increase the levels of pain-suppressing

TABLE 4.1

Antidepressants Commonly Used in Cancer Patients

Drug Name	Brand Name	Daily Dose
Tricyclic antidepressants (TCAs)		
Amitriptyline	Elavil, others	50–300 mg
Amoxapine	Asendin	100–400 mg
Desipramine	Norpramine	50–300 mg
Doxepin	Sinequan	50–300 mg
Imipramine	Tofranil	50–300 mg
Nortriptyline	Pamelor	50–200 mg
Protriptyline	Vivactil	15–60 mg
Trimipramine	Surmontil	50–300 mg
Selective serotonin reuptake inhibitors (SSRIs)		
Fluoxetine	Prozac	10–80 mg
Paroxetine	Paxil	10–50 mg
Sertraline	Zoloft	50–200 mg
Fluvoxamine	Luvox	50–300 mg
Other antidepressants		
Bupropion	Wellbutrin	200–450 mg
Maprotiline	Ludiomil	50–225 mg
Mirtazapine	Remeron	15–45 mg
Nefazodone	Serzone	200–600 mg
Trazodone	Desyrel	150–500 mg
Venlafaxine	Effexor	75–375 mg
Stimulants		
Dextroamphetamine		5–30 mg
Methylphenidate	Ritalin	5–30 mg
Pemoline		30–75

TABLE 4.2

Best Antidepressant Medications for Specific Symptoms

Symptom	Best Choices
Fatigue	Stimulants, fluoxetine (Prozac), sertraline (Zoloft), paroxetine (Paxil)
Insomnia	Trazodone (Desyrel), mirtazapine (Remeron), amitriptyline (Elavil)
Pain	Amitriptyline (Elavil), paroxetine (Paxil)
Opioid side effects	Paroxetine (Paxil), sertraline, (Zoloft), stimulants
Loss of appetite	Paroxetine (Paxil), doxepin (Sinequan), amitriptyline (Elavil)
Anxiety	Paroxetine (Paxil), nortryptiline (Pamelor)

chemicals in the brain, they are sometimes used to treat pain in people who are not depressed.

A lot of different antidepressants are available. Table 4.1 lists some of the most commonly used ones. Your doctor will recommend an antidepressant that is most likely to counteract the most bothersome symptoms of your depression. These are listed in Table 4.2.

Antidepressants can have some side effects. For example, certain antidepressants make you sleepy. If you are having a lot of difficulty sleeping, your doctor will choose one that you can take at bedtime to help you sleep. Other antidepressants can increase appetite, or increase wakefulness and energy. At the same time, the doctor wants to choose an antidepressant without side effects that could make your symptoms worse. These are included in Table 4.3.

Of the three categories of antidepressant medications (see Table 4.1), the tricyclic antidepressants tend to be a bit sedating and increase appetite, so they are often used for persons who are not sleeping or eating well. The tricyclics are also believed to help reduce pain more than the other antidepressants. They have certain side effects, however, that

TABLE 4.3

Side Effects of Commonly Used Antidepressants

Symptom	Sometimes Occurs with	Rarely Occurs with
Agitation/anxiety	All stimulants Bupropion Amoxapine Imipramine Desipramine	Fluoxetine Sertraline Protriptyline
Cardiac arrhythmias	Amitriptyline Amoxapine Imipramine Doxepin Nortriptyline Protriptyline	Desipramine
Dry mouth, urinary or bowel retention	Amitriptyline Doxepin Imipramine Sertraline Paroxetine	Other tricyclics
Headache	Fluoxetine Sertraline	Paroxetine
Hypotension (lower blood pressure) when standing	Amitriptyline Imipramine	Other tricyclics
Increased appetite	Amitriptyline Doxepin Imipramine Desipramine Trimipramine Nortriptyline	Maprotiline
Insomnia	Sertraline Fluoxetine	Paroxetine

Nausea	Fluoxetine	
	Zoloft	
	Paroxetine	
Sedation	Mirtazapine	Amitriptyline
	Doxepin	Amoxapine
	Trazadone	
	Imipramine	
	Desipramine	
	Protriptyline	
	Sertraline	
Sexual dysfunction	Amitriptyline	Imipramine
	Doxepin	
	Amoxipine	
	Desipramine	
	Nortriptyline	
	Protriptyline	
	Trimipramine	

may make them inappropriate for some patients (see Table 4.3). Patients with heart disease, for example, should usually avoid tricyclics, or only take them in low doses.

The serotonin specific antidepressants (SSAs) seem to work more quickly than the tricyclics and are often energizing rather than sedating. They are often selected for persons who are having difficulty staying awake during the day. They cause headaches in a few people, however, and may worsen nausea in some others (see Table 4.3). The other antidepressants have different side effects and are generally used less frequently than the two major types.

A short treatment course with a single antidepressant may be all that is needed, but in many cases, doctors combine two or more medications. Combination therapy can allow lower doses of each medication to be used, lessening the chances of side effects. It may also allow the doctor to use the different side effects to advantage. For example, a person may take an energizing antidepressant, such as fluoxetine, in the morning and a sedating one, such as amitriptyline, at bedtime.

Whatever antidepressant is chosen, it is important to know that it usually takes a few weeks before the medicine works well. Some improvement, particularly with pain, sleeping, and appetite, may occur much sooner.

One other class of medications, the stimulants, are sometimes used to treat depression in cancer patients. The stimulants are rarely, if ever, used to treat other people with depression. Stimulants are not effective in physically healthy people with depression, but they seem to have different effects in people who are chronically ill, or who are taking large doses of opioids (pain medications). Many cancer patients obviously fit both these criteria. In such patients, the stimulants often improve mood, appetite, and concentration, while at the same time lessening feelings of weakness and fatigue. They may also combat feelings of sedation or drowsiness caused by pain medications.

Stimulants can have a significant number of side effects and are, of course, habit-forming. Side effects include increased anxiety, sleeplessness, blood pressure or heart problems, and tremors. In the low doses usually prescribed for cancer patients, however, these side effects are minimal. Tolerance to the stimulants may develop over time, so that a larger dose of the medication will be necessary to get the same effect. Although any of the stimulants can be effective, pemoline is used frequently because it seems to have fewer side effects. It can also be dissolved under the tongue, making it a good choice for people who have difficulty swallowing.

Anxiety

Like depression, some symptoms of tension or anxiety occur in most people with cancer. They are perfectly normal, but can sometimes cause as much interference with daily living as depression does. It is less clear if anxiety actually worsens pain the way that depression does, but there is some evidence that it may do so, at least in certain cases. Muscle pain, which some patients experience after certain types of chemotherapy, is certainly worsened by anxiety, as are headaches.

Anxiety occurs to varying degrees in cancer patients. It often becomes more severe as the disease progresses or as treatment becomes more intense. Almost half of all cancer patients report some anxiety, and about 20 percent have severe or long-lasting anxiety problems. When anxiety becomes severe, it can cause intense fear, difficulty remembering or thinking, and even physical symptoms like shortness of breath, sweating, lightheadedness, and rapid heartbeat. Here is a list of common symptoms of severe anxiety that cancer patients may experience. Note that some of these symptoms, especially numbers 3, 4, 5, and 12, can also be caused by worsening medical conditions. Don't assume a symptom is caused simply by anxiety until you've been evaluated by your doctor for medical problems.

1. Feeling shaky, jittery, or nervous.
2. Feeling tense, fearful, or apprehensive.
3. Feeling your heart pounding or racing.
4. Having trouble catching your breath when nervous.
5. Feeling as if your stomach is tied in knots.
6. Feeling a lump in your throat.
7. Finding yourself pacing, or having trouble sitting still.
8. Worrying about the next diagnostic test or treatment weeks in advance.
9. Being afraid of losing control or going crazy.
10. Obsessively worrying about when your pain will return and how bad it will get.
11. Spending more time in bed because you fear the pain will intensify if you move about.
12. Feeling confused or disoriented, or having difficulty remembering.

Patients who have a tumor involving the brain or lung and those whose chemotherapy includes corticosteroids are more likely to have problems with anxiety. Other factors that may cause anxiety are listed below.

Poorly Controlled Pain

Abnormal Metabolic States
- hypoxia (low oxygen)
- pulmonary embolus (blood clot to the lungs)
- infection
- delirium (impaired mental function and memory)
- hypoglycemia (low blood sugar)
- heart failure
- shortness of breath from any cause, including lung tumor

Hormone-Secreting Tumors
- pheochromocytoma
- thyroid adenoma or carcinoma
- parathyroid adenoma
- pituitary and brain tumors
- insulinoma
- pancreatic cancer

Anxiety-Producing Drugs
- corticosteroids (cortisone, prednisone, Decadron, etc.)
- thyroxine (thyroid hormone supplement)
- bronchodilators
- stimulants
- antihistamines
- benzodiazepines (a paradoxical reaction sometimes seen in the elderly)

Substance Withdrawal (from alcohol, narcotic analgesics, or sedatives)

Anxiety that interferes with the cancer patient's quality of life should be evaluated and treated. When anxiety is caused by a medical situation, such as poorly controlled pain or a hormone-secreting tumor, treating the underlying condition usually controls the anxiety symptoms. Other people find their anxiety is largely relieved as their questions are answered and they are reassured about their condition. Psychotherapy, family therapy, self-help groups, and techniques like hypnosis, meditation, guided imagery, or biofeedback can also be very effective.

As is the case with depression, some people will take an extra pain pill or two to treat spells of anxiety. The biggest problem with doing this is that pain pills are not very effective at treating anxiety; they simply sedate the person taking them. Any of a dozen antianxiety medications (commonly called tranquilizers) do a much better job at treating anxiety without making the person taking them sedated and sleepy. An anxiolytic medication can be used alone or in addition to psychological or self-help techniques. As with symptoms of depression, your doctors may not ask if you are anxious; they expect you to let them know if you are. There are different side effects associated with the different antianxiety medications, but the side effects are generally very mild.

The choice of an antianxiety medication is largely made by the duration of action best suited to the patient. The short-acting benzodiazepines (alprazolam and lorazepam) are effective for intermittent anxiety and panic attacks. Longer acting medications, such as diazepam, are better when there is a constant level of anxiety. One antianxiety medication, buspirone, also has antidepressant effects and may be appropriate for people who are both anxious and depressed. Patients with hormonal or brain tumors that cause their anxiety may not respond well to the usual tranquilizers, but often get relief from "neuroleptic" tranquilizers such as haloperidol or respiridone.

All antianxiety medications can be habit-forming if taken for a long period of time. Most doctors prescribe them on an as-needed basis, up to three or four times a day. If you are not feeling anxious or nervous, it's fine to skip a dose of antianxiety medication. If you have been taking the medication regularly and now feel better, you might want to try tapering off or stopping it every few weeks. However, once you have taken antianxiety medicines regularly for more than a month, do not stop suddenly. Your doctor can help you taper the medicines quite easily, but stopping them suddenly might cause problems.

Anxiety About Pain

For a few people, the major source of anxiety comes from worrying about pain and pain medications. Some people have had a bad experience in the past when they did not get enough pain medication from a doctor when they really needed it. Others are simply terrified that a procedure or treatment will leave them in severe pain. In the past, some doctors were so concerned about patients becoming addicted to pain medication that they often did not prescribe enough to take care of the patient's pain.

Fortunately, that thinking is largely a thing of the past, especially for doctors who work regularly with cancer patients. Even if routine pain medications do not work, there are many alternative treatments that can relieve the pain. If for any reason your oncologist is having trouble controlling your pain, she can refer you to a pain specialist.

Insomnia

Difficulty sleeping is reported by most cancer patients at some point during treatment. Stress and anxiety, nausea from chemotherapy, the effects of medications taken to treat the cancer, and changes in lifestyle can all contribute to insomnia. For many people, the problem is minor and only affects them occasionally. For others, insomnia becomes a significant problem.

One of the major reasons people have trouble sleeping at night is that they have slept during the day. Many people become so drowsy from pain medication that they doze several times a day, and then find that they are not sleepy at bedtime. Others take long naps because they are fatigued from chemotherapy or from not sleeping the night before. Since people often stop work or other activities during a course of chemotherapy, they can sleep later each morning. This often leads to staying up late at night, until eventually the night-day cycle becomes reversed.

Sleeping pills can definitely help to restore normal sleep at night. All sleeping pills are not the same, however. The most commonly used sleeping pills are from the class of medications called benzodiazepines, the same group that includes the most common kinds of tranquilizers. These medications are very effective at first, but over time they often become less and less effective. More importantly, they can cause rebound insomnia. This occurs when someone has taken one of these medications nightly for several weeks or more. After stopping the medications, the insomnia becomes worse than it was before starting. For this reason, most doctors recommend that you do not take this type of sleeping pill every night and do not take it for longer than a month or so.

Other sleeping pills that are not from the benzodiazepine class do not always work quite as well, but they do have several advantages. For the most part, these medications are not habit-forming, and they do not cause tolerance (loss of effect over time) or rebound insomnia. Some of them also result in more natural sleep patterns than do the benzodiazepines. For example, several of the antidepressants cause quite a bit of drowsiness and are effective when used as sleeping pills. Amitriptyline, doxepin, trazodone, and other antidepressants are often prescribed for this purpose. One of the newer antidepressants, mirtazapine (Remeron), is claimed to be particularly effective when used as a sleeping pill.

Many over-the-counter medications and herbal preparations can also help restore normal sleep. The antihistamine medication diphenhydramine (Benadryl) is sold without a prescription as cold pills and sleeping aids under many different brand names. It makes most people quite drowsy and can therefore be used as a sleeping pill.

The hormone melatonin is another sleeping aid sold without a prescription in drug and health food stores. It is often effective by itself, or it may be taken in addition to other sleeping medications. Melatonin does have some hormonal effects, however, so you should check with your oncologist before taking it. Several herbal preparations are claimed to help restore sleep. Some of them may be effective, and all appear to be safe to use.

It is also important not to just depend on medications, but to do other things to help your body return to a normal sleep cycle. When daytime sleepiness is a problem, an energizing type of antidepressant or stimulant may help maintain wakefulness during the day. Setting the alarm clock and getting up at the same time each morning is important for those who are having difficulty falling asleep at night. Avoiding caffeine for at least six hours before bedtime is extremely important for anyone having difficulty sleeping. Remember that most soft drinks and teas have just as much caffeine as coffee does. Some over-the-counter pain and headache remedies also contain caffeine.

Pain Medications and Addiction

At first glance, this topic might not seem to belong in a chapter about factors that make pain worse. However, patient and family (and sometimes physician) fears about addiction have led many people to worry about pain medications, or even to suffer rather than take them.

There is a fairly common myth, believed by some doctors as well as much of the general public, that simply taking opioid (narcotic) medications will create addiction. The origins of this myth began in the days when anyone could buy opium and laudanum. It became apparent that people who frequently took opium or laudanum often became drug addicts. After the world wars, the Korean conflict, and Vietnam, many soldiers came home from overseas addicted to opioids, and the common belief was that they had become addicted because they took morphine for their wounds.

That there is an association between taking opioids and becoming addicted to them no one questions. However, that does not mean there is a cause-and-effect relationship, meaning that doing one thing causes another. Millions of people have taken opioids for an extended time, but only a small fraction of them became drug addicts. There is some evidence that many of those who did become addicted were generally at risk for addiction, whether to opiods or some other substance.

Put in another way, it would be pretty meaningless to say, "We studied alcoholics, and they all drink too much alcohol. Therefore, drinking alcohol will make a person alcoholic." All adults in America can drink alcohol if they wish. The vast majority drink responsibly and never have a problem with it. Many never drink at all. A very few become alcoholics. America has already experimented with making alcohol illegal (Prohibition in the 1930s). Interestingly, the number of people who drank decreased markedly during Prohibition, but the number of alcoholics did not change much. Those addicted to alcohol were still able to get it.

We now understand a lot more about the phenomena of addiction than we did even a decade ago. In order to discuss it we will need to define a few terms. *Addiction* is defined as "continuing to abuse a substance despite repeated adverse consequences." Addiction is associated with dependence, craving, and tolerance. *Tolerance* occurs when more of a drug or medication is needed to get the same effect that a small amount could once give. *Dependence* is when unpleasant symptoms will occur if the medication or drug is stopped suddenly. *Craving* is the emotional and mental obsession with obtaining the substance in order to experience the feeling it creates.

It is important to understand that physical dependence is not addiction. Everyone who takes enough opioids for a long enough time will become physically dependent on them. This simply means they will suffer withdrawal symptoms if they stop the medications suddenly. Opioid withdrawal is not nearly as severe as it is portrayed on television. Most people who have been through it say it's a lot like having the flu. Physical dependence also occurs with a number of medications that are not addictive, such as blood pressure medications.

Of course, doctors do not let their patients go through withdrawal. If someone becomes physically dependent on opioids, we can taper off the medications so that there are no withdrawal symptoms. Opioid tapering is actually done quite often. Most people who have required pain medication for a major surgery probably developed some physical dependence within a week or so of the surgery. However, as pain decreases, the doctor will give less potent and less frequent medications, and the patient will slowly and automatically taper off all medication. Very few of these patients ever experience any withdrawal symptoms, although many would have if the medications had been stopped abruptly a week or two after surgery.

Many cancer patients will become tolerant or physically dependent on their pain medications. Only a very small percentage (most studies say less than 5 percent; many studies say less than 1 percent) will avoid developing the other symptoms of addiction. That is, they do not develop cravings for their pain medications, and they do not continue to use too much of it despite experiencing adverse consequences. Those patients whose cancer is cured can easily taper off the medication when that is appropriate. Tolerance can be overcome by changing the type of pain medication used and the route by which it is administered.

Concerns about addiction to opioids can be real for people who are recovering from a previous addictive disorder or alcoholism. Such people can still take pain medications safely, although it is important their physician understands both addictive disease and pain control. Methadone, which is often used to help opioid addicts overcome addiction, has excellent pain-relieving qualities and can often be very effective for recovering persons who have cancer.

PART II

Standard Treatments for Cancer Pain

CHAPTER 5

Opioid (Narcotic)
Pain Medications

by Daniel Brookoff, M.D.

I t is well recognized that many (although not all) types of cancer can cause pain. This may range from mild muscle aches following chemotherapy to severe pain that markedly interferes with the enjoyment of life. About two-thirds of cancer patients believe they will die in horrible pain. Almost half worry about pain on a daily basis.

There was a time when cancer patients sometimes had to suffer severe pain, but that time is past. Today, more than 95 percent of cancer patients report that their pain is well controlled and does not interfere with their daily lives. Most pain doctors believe that given proper treatment and support, pain could be controlled in virtually every single cancer patient.

The World Health Organization has presented a ladder of pain management for patients with cancer. Patients with minimal pain begin with nonsteroidal anti-inflammatory medications, such as Motrin, for pain control. If this does not control the pain, they take an opioid medication (any medication chemically related to morphine). There are a number of different opioids, some obtained from natural sources (such as morphine and codeine) and others synthesized in the laboratory (such as Stadol and Demerol). They all have generally similar effects, but differ in potency, duration of action, and side effects.

Treating cancer pain with opioids begins as a routine trial. Most cancer doctors use several of these medications frequently and have favorites that they commonly try first. Many patients respond well to the first opioid tried, but some will have side effects, or the first medication may not be strong enough. A few people will have to try several different opioids before they find the one(s) that works best for them.

About Pain and Treatment

With all the treatments for pain discussed in this part, it is important that the patient and doctor work in partnership. This means the patient must have at least a general understanding of what is causing the pain and how the various treatments work. The patient may also need to understand how the doctor thinks about pain and pain treatment. In almost every case, an active patient gets better treatment more rapidly, not because doctors do not care about all patients, but because the knowledgeable, active patient can explain his pain in a way the doctor can understand. With this in mind, we will briefly summarize some of the facts about pain discussed earlier in the book and present some ways you can help your doctor treat your pain more effectively.

Normal Pain and Abnormal Pain

The ability to sense pain is a vital bodily function. Normal pain (often called acute, meaning sudden) is the sensation that something is damaging the tissues of the body. Acute pain is an important alarm that can warn a person of threatened or ongoing injury. Without the sensation of acute pain, we would quickly lose body parts to trauma or would become desperately ill before we sought medical attention. People with acute pain show signs of nervous system activation such as a high heart rate, sweating, and hyperalertness. Their pain is meaningful, has a well-defined cause, and is often reversible. This is the common picture of pain that most patients and physicians carry in their minds.

Cancer patients suffer a chronic pain that is not a normal, useful pain. Whereas acute pain helps warn people of possible injury and helps preserve life, chronic pain serves no useful purpose and stops people from living their lives. It is also quite a different sensation than acute pain and has different effects on the body. Patients with unrelieved cancer pain do not look like patients with normal pain. Instead, they often appear listless or depressed. Because they do not conform to the usual picture of pain, people with cancer pain sometimes do not get appropriate treatment for their pain.

In recent years, the chronic pain associated with cancer has been recognized as a medical illness, in and of itself, that has significant negative effects on health. Uncontrolled pain slows healing, interferes with therapies for medical problems, and even endangers life. Among cancer patients, uncontrolled pain has long been recognized as an important contributing factor to depression and suicide. In other words, cancer pain itself is a dangerous disease that should be treated as aggressively as any other serious medical illness.

Sources of Pain

There are at least three distinct types of pain suffered by people with cancer: somatic, visceral, and neuropathic. (For a more detailed discussion, see chapter 1.) Somatic pain is what most people think of as "normal" pain. Somatic pain originates in skin, muscle, and bone. It is usually well localized and described in unemotional terms (such as sharp, stinging, or aching). This type of pain is related to damage or disruption of tissues such as from a burn, incision, or other injury that damages the tissues. Somatic pain is usually worst at the time of the injury or soon afterward and rapidly tapers off. Doctors feel comfortable treating somatic pain, largely because it is the type of pain they have the most experience with.

Visceral pain refers to pain generated in the internal organs (medically called the viscera, hence visceral pain). The viscera generate pain signals in response to inflammation, distension, or increased pressure but not to incisions or lacerations like somatic tissues. This was demonstrated as long ago as 1628 by Sir William Harvey, the physician to the king of England. Sir William was asked to care for a young boy who had suffered a catastrophic injury to his chest in a riding accident. The injury left the boy's heart and lungs exposed, but he remained able to speak and respond. Sir William noted that if he pricked the boy's skin with his dagger, the boy felt pain. However, the boy did not complain of pain when the dagger pierced his heart or lung. Stretching the lung caused severe pain, however. (Obviously, the ethics of medical experimentation have changed somewhat since Sir William's day.)

The occurrence of visceral pain does not necessarily mean there has been a visceral injury. Most people have experienced the severe, cramping pain that occurs when the bowel is distended by gas, for example. Visceral pain also differs from somatic pain in that it is not well localized. When you cut a finger, you know exactly which finger is cut. When you have visceral pain, you know generally where it hurts, but you could not say, "The right lobe of my liver is painful today." Visceral pain also is often referred to other locations. For example, angina pain from the heart can radiate to the jaw or the left arm. This sometimes makes it difficult to decide where the pain is originating.

A very important fact about visceral pain is that it causes different responses in the brain than somatic pain does. Visceral pain produces stronger autonomic (regulation of the body's functions) responses. For example, visceral pain is more likely to change blood pressure or make you sweat suddenly than is somatic pain. Visceral pain is also associated with stronger emotional responses than comparable somatic pain. The increased emotional content that patients suffering visceral pain experience is a physical characteristic of the pain. It is not due to the person's personality or mental toughness.

A third type of pain, neuropathic pain, is commonly a part of cancer pain. Neuropathic pain is usually caused by damage to nerves. In patients who do not have cancer, neuropathic pain occurs with zoster (shingles), diabetic neuropathy, and some types of nerve damage. After the injury, some fibers in the nerve form abnormal connections while others stop working entirely. The abnormal connections can cause a stimulus that should not be painful (light touch, for example) to become very painful. The patient with neuropathic pain may also experience the pain as a shooting, burning, or electrical shock sensation. At the same time, certain sensations in the area may be lost. This can result in an area being both numb and painful.

Neuropathic pain can be especially agonizing. It does not respond well to opioid medications, so very high doses of pain medications may be needed to provide relief. Neuropathic pain often responds to other types of drugs, however, such as those used to treat seizures (anticonvulsants) or abnormal heart rhythms (antiarrhythmics).

The Body's Ability to Suppress Pain

The body has a very complicated system of nerve pathways to carry pain signals from the organs and tissues to the spinal cord and eventually to the brain. Another complex set of nerve pathways is devoted to turning pain off. This natural pain-relieving system is just as vital to normal functioning as the pain-sensing system. When a pain signal is received in the brain, chemicals called endorphins are released, which send a signal down to the spinal cord, reducing the pain.

For example, if someone smashes her finger with a hammer, she will usually feel intense somatic pain immediately after the injury. This pain signal could be so overwhelming that it dramatically affects her emotions, changing her normal behavior. For example, she might say things she would never say under normal circumstances. Within minutes of the injury, however, the pain usually subsides and she returns to a more normal emotional state. This did not happen because the wound has healed—that would take days. It happened because the pain-relieving system of the body became activated. If it were not for this natural pain-relieving system, many of us would walk around cursing and suffering all the time.

When the natural pain-relieving mechanisms are not enough to control pain, we reduce the pain by using medications that are chemically similar to the natural endorphins of the body. These medications work by stimulating the same receptors in the nervous system (called opioid receptors) that the natural endorphins do. These medications are medically referred to as opioid medications, although many people refer to them as narcotic medications.

Most physicians prefer the term *opioids* because it does not have the negative connotation associated with the term *narcotics*. (As a friend of mine likes to say, "The Mafia sells narcotics. Doctors concerned about pain prescribe opioids.") Opioid medications are the mainstays of treatment for moderate to severe cancer pain and, when used appropriately, can restore the quality of life that has been lost to pain.

The Ethics of Pain Treatment

Medical training, which places a strong emphasis on curing disease, can sometimes lead doctors to reduce their attentions to patients who cannot be cured. This sometimes applies to terminal cancer patients. It may even apply to those whose cancer has been cured, but who are left with long-term pain from the effects of the disease (and sometimes the treatment). However, it is important to remember that even though there may not be a curative treatment for a person's cancer, there will almost always be an effective treatment available for the pain.

Using current treatments, cancer pain can be well controlled in more than 95 percent of patients. With the current understanding of pain and its treatment, doctors should recognize that to leave a patient to suffer with treatable pain is a breach of their ethics as caregivers. Unfortunately, physician training, until the last decade, taught physicians to be absolutely certain a patient had no alternative before prescribing opioid medications.

Today, we realize that opioid medications can be taken on a long-term basis when needed and in higher doses than were considered safe, even in the 1980s. The U.S. Agency for Health Care Policy and Research (AHCPR) has stated that all patients with severe pain should be given opioid medications in sufficient doses to control pain twenty-four hours a day. It has also stated that federal and state policies should never hamper the ability of cancer patients to obtain sufficient opioids to control their pain.

Helping Your Doctor to Treat Your Pain by Giving Accurate Information

The evaluation of chronic pain can be difficult and time consuming for your physician. Most cancer patients are treated by a medical or surgical oncologist who focuses primarily on treating the cancer. The oncologist may simply not have enough time to carefully go through all the symptoms and possible causes of the pain. Most people do not require a thorough pain evaluation, anyway. They have straightforward somatic pain that responds readily to opioid medications.

A patient with more difficult pain problems, however, may experience significant frustration because his pain treatment is not successful. As the pain continues, other important features of the patient's life, such as relationships with family members, become affected. In such cases, a referral to a pain specialist may be an option. Many times, however, if the patient can accurately explain his symptoms to his primary doctor, the doctor will be able to treat the pain effectively.

This sounds simple, but it requires a significant effort on the patient's part. Most people just tell the doctor they hurt in a certain location and how severe the pain is. The doctor, who is trying to determine what is causing the pain and what the most effective treatment would be, needs a lot more information than this. Medically, knowing the characteristics of the pain and how the pain varies at different times and with different activities provides far more important information than simply knowing how severe the pain is. There are several simple things you can do to help your doctor evaluate your pain more accurately.

Be able to report your symptoms accurately.
Keeping a pain diary (a daily record of how severe the pain is each hour) can help. You can rate the severity of pain from one to ten every hour during the day and note in the diary what medications or other pain-relieving things you did. Also note activities such as eating or exercise. The diary can help identify factors that can be treated and also provides information about the cause of the pain itself. Most people who keep a pain diary are very surprised to find that

their pain is more severe at certain times of the day. The diary will also show how well the medication you are taking relieves your pain and how long it lasts.

Include reports of your functional status.
The first thing that patients in pain stop doing are the important activities that are carried on outside work, such as going to church, spending time in family activities, or taking part in hobbies. In some cases of successful treatment, patients will increase their activities as soon as they get any relief, even if this means their overall pain level remains high. If they simply report their pain level, the doctor may not realize that the treatment has helped somewhat. Telling the doctor that you have been able to function better may prevent her from abandoning the treatment too soon.

Accurately report all medications you take,
including over-the-counter medicine.
Many people think that over-the-counter medicine or herbal preparations somehow don't count. This is not the case at all. For example, many people are taking over-the-counter pain relievers that contain acetaminophen (Tylenol). Since many prescription pain pills also contain acetaminophen, an overdose could occur if these were given. An acetaminophen overdose can cause liver failure.

Report the characteristics of the pain.
The most important help you can give to the doctor is an accurate description of the symptoms or type of pain you are experiencing. This can be difficult to do, but can greatly aid your doctor in identifying the source of your pain. Below is a list of adjectives you might use to describe your pain:

- Throbbing
- Pounding
- Shooting
- Stabbing
- Electrical shock
- Cramping

- Gnawing
- Burning
- Pressure
- Itching
- Dull
- Sharp

- Aching
- Heavy
- Tender
- Splitting
- Tingling

Here is a list of symptoms you might describe to your doctor that may be associated with the pain:

- Sweating all over
- Sweating in one part of the body
- Feeling hot or flushed
- Rapid pulse
- Dizziness
- Numbness
- Pounding in head
- Feeling faint or passing out

- Nausea
- Butterflies in stomach
- Churning or cramps in stomach
- Difficulty swallowing
- Dry mouth
- Muscles aching, twitching, or jumping
- Tension in jaw muscles
- Skin crawling or itching

Do not exaggerate or dramatize.

Sometimes people feel they have to impress a doctor with how severe the pain is. Other times, the frustration of being in pain pours out during the few minutes they spend with the doctor. Getting too dramatic or emotional is almost guaranteed to backfire, however. Remember that every doctor has seen injuries and damage to the body you may not be able to imagine. As soon as you say, "No one can imagine how bad my pain is," the doctor remembers about one hundred people who certainly did have worse pain. Weeping, moaning, or threatening suicide may simply convince the doctor you are depressed or hysterical, rather than making any impression about your pain. A simple, factual explanation about how the pain interferes with your life is much more likely to be helpful.

Describe the intensity of the pain.

This information is most important to the doctor. The pain intensity influences the selection of medication, the route of administration, and the rate of dose adjustment. It is important for the doctor to know about, particularly as he tries different medications to help the pain.

Setting Goals

It is important to develop a set of goals in collaboration with your doctor to guide treatment and assess progress. At first, these may be very simple, such as being able to spend an afternoon out with the family or being able to sleep through the night. With time, the goals may get more complicated, such as returning to work or enjoying recreational activities. This approach involves determining what things are missing from your life that you wish to restore.

The medical evaluation of cancer pain must be comprehensive enough to yield effective strategies for dealing with *all* the sources of the pain. This certainly includes a thorough medical evaluation, but may often include psychological and social evaluations. A complete assessment of chronic pain means developing an appreciation for how pain has invaded the patient's life and contributed to changes in behavior, attitudes, and relationships. The goal of pain treatment is to enable the patient to reclaim that life.

Using Opioid Medications to Treat Cancer Pain

For nearly every case of severe cancer pain, there is a treatment that will result in quick, effective, and safe pain relief. Every person is different, however, and sometimes the doctor may have to try several different medications to find a combination that effectively relieves your pain without causing side effects.

Opioid medications are the primary pain-relieving (or analgesic) medications used for the treatment of moderate to severe cancer pain. When used properly, these medications reduce the abnormal pain without impairing the body's ability to feel normal pain. People using opioid medications can get excellent relief from cancer pain, but will still feel pain if they stub a toe or cut a finger.

The strategy used to treat chronic pain is different from that used to treat the acute pain that follows surgery or injury. For acute pain, short-acting medications are given on an as-needed basis. In this approach,

TABLE 5.1

Dose Equivalents for Opioid Analgesics

Doses are equivalent to 10 mg of injected morphine. Medications are listed in order of increasing potency.

Drug	Approximate Dose		Dosage Interval
	Oral	*Injected*	
Codeine*	180–200 mg	60 mg	3–4 hours
Meperidine (Demerol)	300 mg	100 mg	3 hours
Morphine	45 mg	10 mg	3–4 hours
Morphine (time-release) (MS Contin)	90–120 mg	N/A	8–12 hours
Hydrocodone (Vicodin, etc.)	30 mg	10 mg	3–4 hours
Oxycodone (Percodan, etc.)	30 mg	10 mg	3–4 hours
Oxycodone (time-release) (Oxycontin)	60 mg	N/A	8–12 hours
Methadone (Dolophine)	20 mg	10 mg	6–8 hours
Hydromorphone (Dilaudid)	7.5 mg	1.5 mg	3–4 hours
Levorphanol (Levodromoran)	4 mg	2 mg	6–8 hours
Oxymorphone (Numorphan)	1 mg	1 mg	3–4 hours

Codeine cannot be given in higher doses because of side effects.

pain medications are used only when the pain occurs. This strategy is not recommended for patients with chronic cancer pain because it will guarantee periods of pain and anxiety. For chronic cancer pain, long-acting medications are used to prevent as much pain as possible with fast-acting medications added as needed for episodes of increased pain.

There are a variety of opioid medications listed in Table 5.1 available for treating cancer pain. The selection of the best one for an individual depends on the type of pain experienced and the person's overall medical conditions. However, the effects and side effects of the various opioids vary slightly in different individuals. For this reason, it is common to try several of these medications before finding one that works best for you. One doctor should take responsibility for pain treatment, and all prescriptions for pain medications should come from that physician. A complete record of each medication's effectiveness and side effects can then be kept, helping you to find the best medicine quickly.

The following paragraphs discuss some commonly used opioid medications. They are listed by their generic names, with some of the more common brand names in parentheses. Generally, the long-acting (either controlled-release or naturally long-acting) opioids are used to manage constant pain, with shorter acting medication added for episodes of more severe pain. The medications are also listed in Appendix A.

Opioid Medications with Controlled-Release Forms

These medications are naturally short acting (their effects last from a few minutes to three or four hours) but are available in time-release, long-acting forms that can last from eight to seventy-two hours per dose. Because of this, a patient can take a controlled-release form for regular pain and a short-acting form of the same medication as a fast-onset "rescue" medication for episodes of increased pain. Note that many of these controlled-release medications are quite expensive. If medication cost is important, the long-acting opioids discussed in the next part may provide an effective alternative.

Morphine (*Controlled release:* MS-Contin, Cadian, Oramorph. *Immediate release:* MS-IR, Roxanol)
Morphine is a naturally occurring (obtained from the opium poppy) opioid thought of as the standard medication for severe cancer pain, probably because it was the first medication used for this purpose. Morphine was also the first opioid to be manufactured in a controlled-release form in the United States in 1984. Because most cancer physicians are very familiar with controlled-release morphine, it is often the first opioid prescribed for severe pain.

Because it has been available longer than other controlled-release formulations, morphine is available in slightly less expensive generic brands. MS-Contin and Oramorph-SR are given every eight or twelve hours. Cadian may last up to twenty-four hours, but usually is given every twelve hours. Cadian has an additional advantage; in powder form it can be sprinkled on soft foods for those who cannot swallow a capsule.

Unlike the controlled-release capsules, the short-acting forms of morphine are very inexpensive. They are available in tablets (morphine sulfate), capsules (MS-IR), liquid (Roxanol), and suppositories.

Oral morphine has a slower onset of action than other oral opioid medications. The controlled-release forms may not have a strong effect for one or two hours after a dose. Morphine is associated with more nausea, itching, and hives than the other opioids. Morphine should not be used by patients who have impaired kidney function.

Fentanyl (*Controlled release:* Duragesic. *Immediate release:* Actiq)
Fentanyl is a synthetic (manufactured in a laboratory) opioid that was first introduced as an alternative to morphine in 1960. For the first thirty years after its release, fentanyl was only available in an injectable form and was used primarily as an anesthetic. It cannot be made into an oral medication because the liver breaks it down so quickly that it is not effective when taken by mouth. In 1990, fentanyl was introduced in a skin patch (Duragesic) that delivers a steady level of medication for up to seventy-two hours.

It takes the duragesic patch about six hours to start working, and twelve to twenty-four hours to reach complete effectiveness. Fentanyl is deposited in the skin, so the medication continues to enter the body for about six hours after the patch is removed. Because of this, once the patch has been started, the level of medication remains very steady, even when changing to a new patch.

The ability to control pain while only having to take a medication every seventy-two hours can dramatically improve quality-of-life for patients with cancer pain. The fentanyl patch has the advantage of being useful for people who cannot take their medications orally. Because the medication is absorbed through the skin and not through the gastrointestinal tract, the fentanyl patch causes less constipation than other controlled-release opioids. It may also improve sleep for cancer pain patients because of the steadiness of the drug levels.

The drug's rate of release can be accelerated if the patient has a high fever (temperature higher than 103°F), and this may require removal of the patch. Some people react to the adhesive in the patch and develop a localized skin rash where the patch has been placed. This can be prevented by pretreating the skin with a steroid spray, such as the kind used in asthma inhalers.

Since 1998, fentanyl has also been available in a fast-acting form called an orulet, which is a flavored lozenge on a stick, similar to a lollipop. This form of fentanyl (Actiq) is placed inside the cheek, where it is rapidly absorbed directly into the bloodstream (often within fifteen seconds), making it very useful against episodic pain. The orulet is left in the mouth for fifteen minutes; its pain-relieving effects can last one to two hours.

Oxycodone (*Controlled release:* OxyContin. *Immediate release:* Oxy-IR, Percocet, Percodan, Roxicet, Roxicodone, Endocet, Tylox)
Oxycodone is a synthetic opioid that is 50 percent more potent than morphine at the same dose. Until recently, it was only available in a short-acting, low-dosage form (such as Percocet, Tylox), so it was generally thought of as a medium-strength opioid. Since 1994, it has been available as a long-acting medication (OxyContin) that is given every eight or twelve hours.

Because many physicians and patients had experience with the short-acting form, they were comfortable using the long-acting form for chronic pain. OxyContin is now the most commonly used controlled-release opioid in the United States. It is designed to deliver up to a third of its contents in the first hour and then to slowly release the remainder over eight to twelve hours. Because of this, it has a much quicker onset of action than the other sustained-release medications. This may explain the increase in side effects that sometimes occurs when patients are taking high doses of this medication.

Oxycodone is a pro-drug, which means it must be metabolized by the liver to become active. Up to 8 percent of the population is deficient in the enzyme needed to initiate this activation. Medications that interfere with this enzyme (including some antidepressants such as Prozac and Paxil) can reduce the effectiveness of oxycodone. Oxycodone generally has fewer gastrointestinal side effects than morphine. The short-acting forms of oxycodone are usually manufactured in combination with acetaminophen (Percocet, Tylox, Roxicet) or aspirin (Percodan), so patients must be aware that they are taking more than one drug at a time. This can be important when assessing drug interactions or side effects.

Hydromorphone (Pallidone, Dilaudid)

Hydromorphone is a synthetic opioid with the pain-relieving effects of morphine but somewhat fewer side effects. A controlled-release form of this medication, which can be taken every twenty-four hours, should become available in the United States next year. Hydromorphone is commonly used in intravenous pumps and is also available in suppository form. It is often used for breakthrough or episodic pain. Unless it is taken in controlled-release form, hydromorphone is too short acting to use for relieving constant pain.

Long-Acting Opioids

These opioids are naturally long-acting medications that do not require a time-release preparation. Their onset is quick (usually within thirty minutes), and they can have pain-relieving effects for six to eight hours after each dose.

Methadone (Dolophine)

Methadone was first synthesized in Germany at the end of World War II. It was specifically designed for the treatment of severe chronic cancer pain. In the mid-1960s, it became widely used to treat drug addicts because it can suppress drug craving in this population with one daily dose. Because of this, it has a reputation as a medication linked to addiction. Actually, it is an excellent pain medication that probably has lower addiction and abuse potential than the other opioids.

For effective pain treatment, methadone should be taken every six to eight hours. Because it has effects on other receptors (called NMDA receptors) in addition to opioid receptors, methadone is sometimes effective for treating pain that does not respond to other opioids. One of the major advantages of methadone is its low cost, particularly when compared to the time-release opioids, all of which are rather expensive.

One danger that is specific to methadone is delayed-onset sedation. The other opioids cause their strongest sedating effects within the first two or three days of use. Methadone, however, may actually cause more sedation for up to two weeks after beginning steady use. This makes methadone particularly difficult for use with elderly patients.

Many physicians mistakenly think that they cannot legally prescribe methadone without a special license. However, this license is only required if the methadone is being prescribed for maintenance therapy of a narcotic addict. When methadone is prescribed to treat cancer pain, its regulations and restrictions are the same as for any other strong opioid medication.

A long-acting form of methadone, L-alpha-acetylmethadol (LAAM), can last up to ninety-six hours per dose. However, it probably will not be used in this country because of its toxic effects on the heart.

Levorphanol (Levodromoran)
Levorphanol is a very potent opioid medication (approximately five times more potent than morphine) that lasts from four to eight hours. It is very well absorbed orally and generally has fewer side effects than morphine. It is also relatively inexpensive. Like methadone, levorphanol may activate a broader range of opioid receptors than most of the other opioid medications. There is some evidence that it gives superior relief for the treatment of neuropathic pain than the other opioids do.

Short-Acting Opioids

These are all short-acting (three to four hours per dose) medications that are not available in controlled-release forms. For cancer patients, they are usually rescue or breakthrough pain medications.

Codeine (Tylenol #3, Empirin)
Codeine is probably the most commonly prescribed opioid in the world. Since it is a fairly weak medication that lasts for three or four hours, it is most appropriate for mild pain. It is associated with a greater incidence of side effects (especially nausea, hives, and itching) than the other opioids. The liver breaks down 10 percent of an oral dose of codeine to morphine, and this may cause codeine's analgesic effects. Codeine is

uniquely effective for the treatment of cough, even in small doses that do not relieve pain.

Hydrocodone (Lortab, Vicodin, Vicoprofen, Tussionex)

Hydrocodone is very commonly used to treat mild to moderate pain. It is available in several different strengths and is generally effective for three to four hours. It is very similar in effect to oxycodone and requires the same liver enzyme to be activated. Hydrocodone is generally available only in combination with aspirin or acetaminophen.

Meperidine (Demerol, Mepergan, Mepergan-Forte)

In its oral form, meperidine is a very short-lived drug that generally does not last more than two or three hours when used to treat severe pain. One of its breakdown products, normeperidine, can cause euphoria, agitation, and—with prolonged usage—personality changes and epileptic seizures. Normeperidine can remain in the body for more than fifteen hours after every dose.

Normeperidine levels, therefore, will continuously increase whenever meperidine is used steadily for more than three or four days. This effect is even greater in people with kidney problems. For this reason, meperidine is never recommended for the treatment of chronic cancer pain.

Diamorphine (Heroin)

Diamorphine (heroin) is not legally available in the United States and is only mentioned because well-meaning patient advocates are lobbying for its legalization as a pain medication for cancer patients. Heroin is a pro-drug and is devoid of opioid activity. In the body, liver metabolism changes heroin to morphine, which causes its analgesic effects. Heroin is purported to have a slightly quicker onset of action and a slightly greater potency than morphine (although only when injected intramuscularly), but this rarely would provide any advantage in the treatment of cancer pain.

Propoxyphene (Darvon, Darvocet)

Although chemically similar to methadone, propoxyphene is a very weak opioid medication. In some studies, it has not been shown to be any more effective in relieving pain than acetaminophen. At the same time, some patients obtain three to six hours of relief from mild to moderate pain with this medication. There is some evidence that propoxyphene might be more effective in females than in males, but the reason for this is unclear. Propoxyphene generally has fewer side effects than other opioids.

Tramadol (Ultram)

Tramadol is a synthetic pain reliever with weak opioid effects. Because its potential for abuse is thought to be less than the other opioid medications, it is not subject to the same prescribing restrictions as are the controlled opioid medications. It is generally considered less potent than codeine, which is one of the weaker opioids. Nevertheless, tramadol has proven to be effective for some people with mild to moderate pain. Tramadol causes less constipation and sedation than the other opioids but can cause considerable nausea in certain people. It also may have some antidepressant effects.

Starting Treatment with Opioids

Short-Acting Opioids

For the patient who has not been on a steady regimen of opioids before, treatment usually starts with a short-acting opioid (such as oxycodone, hydromorphone, or morphine). When using these short-acting opioids, most patients will require doses every three to six hours. Commonly used medications and starting doses for severe pain include: oxycodone, 10 to 15 mg, codeine, 30 to 60 mg, morphine, 15 to 30 mg, hydromorphone, 2 to 4 mg, or levorphanol, 2 to 4 mg. Most doctors recommend trying the medication for at least forty-eight hours to obtain relief. (Of course, it should be stopped immediately if it causes side effects.)

If the medication is not effective after forty-eight hours, most doctors will try increasing the dose. If this is not effective, then a trial of a different opioid is usually indicated.

It is important to provide your doctor with as much information as possible when the medication does not work. When a medication lessens the pain a little, but not enough to give good relief, simply increasing the dose may be effective. If that helps but does not last long enough, changing to a time-release form may be better.

Long-Acting Opioids

For people with continuous or frequently recurring cancer pain, a time-release opioid preparation can be started once there has been a good response to the short-acting opioid. The most commonly prescribed preparations are long-acting forms of either morphine or oxycodone that allow dosing intervals from eight to twelve hours. The starting daily dose should be roughly equivalent to the total daily consumption of the short-acting medication. The fentanyl patch is also a reasonable long-acting opioid to start out with, once a person has become accustomed to the short-acting medications (i.e., early-onset side effects such as hives or nausea have resolved).

The long-acting medications, such as levorphanol and methadone, can be very useful for treating severe cancer pain, but they are usually reserved as second-line drugs because they are more difficult to adjust and can have delayed side effects. Because of the long-term effects of these medications, they are generally prescribed only for patients who have been using opioids for some time.

No matter which long-acting medication is used, it should be taken on a "by-the-clock" schedule whether the patient is hurting or not. All patients who receive long-acting opioids should also be supplied with a fast-acting rescue drug taken on an as-needed basis to treat pain that breaks through the regular medication schedule. Rescue doses are usually equivalent to between 5 and 15 percent of a daily dose of long-acting opioid. (See Table 5.1.)

Although most doctors will allow rescue medication every two to four hours, patients who require it that frequently probably should have their doses of long-acting medication increased. By observing how much rescue drug a patient requires, the doctor can determine how much the controlled-release drug should be increased. This process is called titration. By titrating the drug dose to the pain, the patient can quickly find a dose of controlled-release medication that provides good relief without causing severe sedation.

There are several important points about titration. First, patients should titrate their medications with their doctor's permission and keep the doctor informed of any changes they make. Most doctors are very agreeable when a patient calls after a day or two asking to increase his medication. By the same token, most are less than receptive when a patient uses a month's worth of medication in ten days without telling the doctor it wasn't working well.

Second, long-acting or time-release opioids should never be taken closely together. These medications may not have their peak effect for several hours after they have been taken. If a second dose of long-acting medication is taken before the first has had an effect, an overdose could occur. Finally, if the medication is having no effect at all, it may not be absorbing properly (see chapter 7), and a different type of medication may be needed.

Selection of Opioids

In selecting the best opioid for chronic cancer pain, it is important to carefully review the medication used previously and any side effects that occurred. Often, a patient will tell the physician of an opioid medication that worked in the past but was used in inadequate doses or inappropriate frequencies. In other cases, some simple trials of several different opioids are needed to find an effective medication that does not cause side effects. In a study of cancer patients requiring opioid medications, 44 percent required trials of two or more medications, and 20 percent required three or more trials before achieving satisfactory pain relief with tolerable side effects. Certain medical considerations also guide the choice of opioid drug. For example, morphine, meperidine, and propoxyphene should not be given to patients with kidney problems.

Sometimes patients do very well at the beginning of treatment with opioids, but find within a few weeks that they are beginning to encounter more pain. This is especially true of patients who severely limited their activities while they were in pain. This is not a sign of tolerance to the medications; it is simply a call for retitration of their dosage. It takes more pain medication to provide comfort for someone undertaking a busy schedule than for someone who is lying in bed all day.

Side Effects of Opioid Medications

One of the most important subjects in managing opioid therapy is controlling or avoiding the side effects of the medications. Many of the side effects of opioids are temporary and will resolve on their own after a week or two of continued use. Some of the commonly encountered temporary side effects include nausea and vomiting, itching, and somnolence.

The one side effect of opioids that generally persists throughout their use is constipation. There is no evidence that opioid medications cause damage to any internal organs, even with prolonged use. Studies have followed people who have steadily used opioids under medical supervision for up to twenty years and have shown that the opioids do not cause any medical problems.

Nausea and Vomiting

Between 10 and 40 percent of patients suffer opioid-induced nausea, particularly when taking higher doses. Nausea can be treated with an antinausea (antiemetic) medication such as promethazine (Phenergan) or prochlorperazine (Compazine), either as pills or suppositories. Patients who are getting good pain relief with an opioid but having problems with nausea can take their antiemetic on a scheduled basis (e.g., four times a day) for a few days until the nausea resolves. If the nausea primarily occurs after eating or if they experience bloating and loss of appetite, metoclopramide (Reglan) may be more effective than standard antinausea medication. For some patients, antihistamines such as hydroxyzine (Vistaril) can also help reduce nausea. Most patients find that the nausea completely resolves within a week to ten days.

Itching and Hives

Some people develop itching and hives when starting an opioid. This is a direct effect of the medication and is usually not an allergic reaction. Itching is more common with the naturally occurring opioids (e.g., codeine, morphine) than with the synthetic medications. Itching and hives are easily relieved with antihistamines. Patients with a previous history of having developed hives or itching with an opioid can use an antihistamine on schedule (three to four times per day) for the first two to three days of therapy. As with nausea, itching usually resolves in a week or so.

Sedation

Opioid medications can sometimes produce sedation or somnolence, though patients with severe pain often feel more alert or more normal while using opioid analgesics. Tolerance to sedation usually develops within days or weeks of taking the medication regularly. If the medication is providing good pain relief, often the best course of action is to limit activities (such as driving, working, preparing meals, taking care of children) until the sedation has passed. If the sedation is not tolerable, try reducing the opioid dose by 25 percent. If sedation persists, but the medication provides effective pain relief, you should ask your doctor if any other medications you are taking might be sedating. Antihistamines, antiemetics, and tranquilizers often add to opioid sedation.

Jerking Movements (Myoclonus)

Myoclonus, or sudden jerking movements of the arms or legs, is sometimes a side effect of opioid use, particularly at bedtime or during the evening. If the problem is severe, it can be treated with a mild benzodiazepine tranquilizer. Clonazepam is a good choice for this problem because it is less sedating than the other benzodiazepine medications.

Constipation

One of the side effects of opioids experienced by most patients is constipation. Unfortunately, patients do not develop tolerance to constipation, and it may worsen when the dose of opioid is increased. It is important for patients taking opioids to prevent constipation rather than trying to treat it after it has become severe. Patients should find a laxative dose they can take nightly that will result in a formed bowel movement every morning. Most doctors recommend taking stool softener (docusate, Colace) every day. Many patients also take a mild fiber-based laxative (senna, Senekot) daily.

If constipation becomes severe, osmotic diuretics, such as milk of magnesia, magnesium citrate, or lactulose (Chronulac), are usually effective. These laxative agents are safe and not habit-forming like the stimulant laxatives. A sodium phosphate enema can also be used. Stimulant laxatives, such as Ex-Lax or Dulcolax, should absolutely be avoided. They are generally not very effective against opioid constipation and in the long term will worsen the problem.

Slowed Breathing (Respiratory Depression)

The most feared side effect of opioids is an overdose causing respiratory depression. If a person in pain is carefully titrated on opioid medications, respiratory depression does not occur. Before the dose of opioid necessary to suppress the respiratory center is reached, the patient has already become unresponsive. This means that a person who is awake and complaining of pain is not in imminent danger of suffering an overdose. Respiratory depression can occur if several doses of opioid are taken before the first has had time to take effect.

It is important for family members to realize that the cancer patient who has taken opioids long term is tolerant to this effect. However, it occasionally happens that a family member "borrows" a pain pill from the cancer patient, sometimes with catastrophic effects.

Swelling (Edema)

Another side effect of the opioid medications is the accumulation of fluid, especially in the feet and hands, caused by opioids stimulating the release of certain hormones. Swelling can usually be treated with diuretics (fluid pills). Speaking of fluids, opioids may also increase the tone of the bladder muscles, causing difficulty urinating. This occurs more commonly in males, especially those with prostate problems.

Tolerance to Opioids

After taking an opioid medication for several weeks or months, some patients will develop tolerance, a reduced effect from a given dose. Tolerance to the unwanted side effects of opioids, such as nausea, is expected. There is controversy over how much tolerance develops to the pain-relieving effects of opioids. Studies of patients on long-term opioids indicate that once pain relief has been obtained, the required dose changes little unless the disease worsens or another source of pain develops. Most of the information we have about opioid tolerance and physical dependence in humans was gained from subjects who were not in pain.

Physical Dependence on Opioids

Physical dependence refers to the physical withdrawal symptoms that can occur when a medication is stopped abruptly. Physical dependence is not limited to opioids; it can happen with a variety of other medications, such as blood pressure medications and steroids. Physical dependence is a medical issue and not a psychological or a spiritual problem.

When the opioid is no longer needed, tapering off the medication can easily manage the physical dependence. This can always be done in an outpatient setting without discomfort for the patient. Often, when cancer treatment begins to work for a patient who has been on opioids, that patient will begin to report sedation on what had been a tolerable opioid dose, or will stop using the rescue medications. When this occurs, it is time to start tapering off the long-acting pain medications. Your doctor can provide a reduced dose of the medication, but most patients find they have no trouble tapering off themselves without medical help.

Note: Some controlled-release medications, particularly OxyContin, should never be broken or cut in half because that interferes with the time-release function. Never cut or break a time-release pill without checking with your doctor or pharmacist.

Agonist-Antagonist Medications

Some opioid medications are referred to as agonist-antagonists. This means the medications partly stimulate the opioid receptors and partly block it. The agonist-antagonists have a ceiling effect; that is, after a certain dose, the antagonist effect begins and giving more of the medication does not create any more pain relief. Agonist-antagonist medications are frequently used by emergency room physicians and some other doctors because the ceiling effect prevents the medications from being abused and minimizes the risk of respiratory depression.

For patients who have been taking potent opioids, an agonist-antagonist medication simply acts to block the potent opioids from the opioid receptor. In simple terms, adding an agonist-antagonist medication actually increases pain. If the patient has been taking potent opioids for a long time, the agonist-antagonist will cause immediate opioid withdrawal. Although no physician would purposely place a cancer patient in withdrawal, some may not be aware of this possibility and might give one of these medications without knowing the consequences. This has also occurred when a cancer patient has "borrowed" someone else's medications hoping to get more relief. Commonly used agonist-antagonist medications include Butorphanol (Stadol), Nalbuphene (Nubain), Pentazocine (Talwin), and Tramadol (Ultram). If you are taking potent opioid medications, you should avoid these medications.

Pseudoaddiction

The fear of drug abuse and drug addiction is the major reason physicians are reluctant to prescribe opioid medications for patients with severe pain. Drug abuse is the inappropriate use of a medication for a non-medical problem. Using a pain medication to attain euphoria or "get high" is inappropriate, as is using drugs to solve family or situational problems that need to be dealt with by other means. The appropriate role of medicine is to prolong and maintain life, promote function, and provide comfort from symptoms of medical problems.

If a person who has been precluded from living life fully by a medical problem (such as physical pain) is using a medication to get back into life, then he is using that medication appropriately. If that patient is using medications to mentally escape from emotional problems (such as family, social, or financial problems), then that patient is abusing drugs.

If taken to the extreme, drug abuse can become the driving force in a person's life, leading to a compulsive pattern of drug abuse and inappropriate or dangerous behaviors. The definition of drug addiction is just that—repeated overuse of a substance despite adverse consequences. If there is a question of abuse, it is up to the physician to determine whether the medications are being used to participate in or to escape from life. The patient's mood and activities and the reports of family members can be helpful indicators.

The medical use of opioids is not associated with the development of addiction. However, inappropriately labeling a cancer patient as an addict can be dangerous. It will alienate the patient from caregivers and family, deepening her isolation and prolonging her suffering. Some cancer patients do become manipulative or obsessive about pain medication, not because they are addicts, but because they do not have good pain control. This constellation of behaviors has been termed pseudoaddiction. Pseudoaddiction can be effectively and legitimately treated by providing adequate pain relief.

Some people, including some physicians who do not understand the issues of chronic pain and the chemical actions of opioids, hold the mistaken belief that opioid medications are inherently bad or dangerous. Opioids are no more or less dangerous than most other medications when used properly under a physician's supervision. As St. Thomas Aquinas said in his book *The Angelic Doctor*, "Nothing is intrinsically good or evil, but its manner of usage may make it so."

CHAPTER 6

Other Medications Used to Treat Cancer Pain

by Daniel Brookoff, M.D.

A lthough opioid medications are a mainstay of cancer pain treatment, a number of other medications can help provide pain relief. The nonsteroidal anti-inflammatory drugs (usually just called nonsteroidals, or NSAIDs) are often used by themselves to treat mild pain. They may be used with opioids, particularly for people who are suffering from bone pain. Antidepressants may also help opioids work better and may have some pain-relieving properties when used alone.

Some of these other medications are actually more effective than opioids in certain situations. Antiseizure medications and benzodiazepines can be more effective for treating nerve pain, for example, than the opioids are. Antispasmodics can relieve certain muscle pains more effectively than other pain medications. Finally, several medications are used as adjuncts (helper medications) in some unusual situations.

This chapter discusses a *lot* of medications, more than any single person will ever use. It is important to cover many medications for two reasons, however. First, if you take one of these classes of medications but are bothered by side effects, or the medicine is not as effective as you would like, you may find an alternative medication that might be substituted. If so, mention it to your doctor to see if it might be appropriate for you. Second, if you are continuing to hurt despite taking opioid medications, you might glance over the different groups of medications. If the description of one group sounds as though they might be helpful, discuss them with your doctor. She may have very good reasons why those medications are not appropriate in your case. On the other hand, you might find something that could be worth trying for your pain.

Nonsteroidal Anti-Inflammatory Medications

Pain that requires medical treatment occurs in 25 percent of patients who are newly diagnosed with cancer, 33 percent of those who are actively undergoing cancer treatment, and up to 75 percent of people with advanced cancers. When treating pain due to cancer, the choice of pain medication sometimes depends more on the intensity of the pain than on the specific type of cancer that is causing it. For mild to moderate pain, the most commonly prescribed medications are the nonsteroidal anti-inflammatory drugs (NSAIDs). These are the medications, such as Motrin and others, that are commonly used to treat headaches, muscle pain, and arthritis. NSAIDs have become the most commonly used pain-relieving medications in the world, especially since they became available over the counter.

Different NSAID Medications

NSAID medications include aspirin, ibuprofen (Motrin, Advil, etc.), naproxen (Aleve, Anaprox, Naprosyn), nabumetone (Relafen), ketoprofen (Orudis), and indomethacin (Indocin). All the NSAIDs are available as oral medications in either tablet or capsule form. For patients who are unable to take oral medications, many of the NSAID medications are available as rectal suppositories. Ketorolac (Toradol) is the only NSAID currently available both in an injectable form (intravenous or intramuscular) and as an oral medication. When ketorolac is injected in high doses, it can sometimes give pain relief comparable to that given by opioid (narcotic) medications.

For most people, any one NSAID medication is as good as any other for the treatment of pain. The most significant variation among the

NSAIDs is in their side effects, so your doctor's first goal is to find one that does not cause you any problems. There are some individual variations in effectiveness, however, probably because the different NSAIDs vary somewhat in how potent their anti-inflammatory effect is in a particular individual.

One feature of using NSAIDs for the treatment of pain is that they have a ceiling effect. This means that beyond a certain dose, increasing the amount of the medication will not yield more pain relief, just more side effects. The ceiling dose may differ for different individuals, but the maximal safe dose of an NSAID is generally two to three times the starting dose. More importantly for cancer patients, the effective pain-relieving doses of the NSAIDs tend to occur at the lower range of the dosing scale. Increasing the dose beyond this point may yield more anti-inflammatory effects, but this does not necessarily give more pain relief. Unlike the opioid (narcotic) pain medications, tolerance and physical dependence do not develop with prolonged use of NSAIDs.

Acetaminophen (Tylenol) selectively blocks the production of prostaglandins in the central nervous system without affecting prostaglandin levels in the organs and tissues. Because of this, acetaminophen is not generally regarded as an anti-inflammatory drug. Nonetheless, acetaminophen is generally as effective for the relief of mild pain and the reduction of fever as are the NSAIDs. It is not as effective as NSAIDs for bone pain or pain associated with inflammation in the tissues, however.

Side Effects of NSAIDs

Stomach Problems

Even though aspirin and other NSAID medications have been used for almost two hundred years, the mechanism by which they work was not discovered until 1971. The NSAIDs all give pain relief and reduce fevers by inhibiting the formation of inflammatory chemicals called prostaglandins (see chapter 1). Prostaglandins, among their other effects, cause pain and inflammation in the tissues and help transmit pain messages in the central nervous system. They are also important in generating the stomach's protective lining, maintaining normal kidney function, and helping the blood to clot.

Suppressing prostaglandin formation can leave the stomach lining unprotected from the effects of stomach acid, resulting in stomach pain, stomach irritation (gastritis), and even the formation of stomach ulcers and bleeding. Much of the stomach irritation due to NSAIDs can be avoided by taking these medications with food. Food in the stomach slows the absorption of NSAID medications slightly, but does not decrease the total amount of medication that is absorbed.

In a few people, especially those with certain risk factors, the use of NSAIDs has caused dangerous stomach hemorrhages requiring hospitalization and transfusions. Having stomach irritation or heartburn does not predict that a person will eventually develop bleeding in his stomach. At the same time, up to two-thirds of people who have gastrointestinal bleeding or ulcers due to NSAIDs had no stomach symptoms before the bleeding or perforation occurred. In other words, stomach pain can occur without ulcers, and ulcers can occur without stomach pain. Here are some factors that put people at high risk for stomach-related side effects from NSAIDS:

- Older than sixty
- History of excess alcohol use
- History of ulcer disease or chronic gastritis
- Using NSAIDs for a long time
- Using steroid medications (cortisone) and NSAIDs together

Whenever a person develops stomach irritation or bleeding due to an NSAID, it is necessary to stop using this type of medication, or at least to change to a different NSAID. If the problem is mild, these side effects can be prevented or treated by using antacids or antiulcer medications (such as Tagamet, Zantac, Prilosec, Prevacid, or Aciphex). Although these drugs are often used to protect the stomach from NSAIDs, their effectiveness for this specific purpose has never been conclusively proven.

Misoprostol (Cytotec) is a medication that has been proven to specifically protect the stomach lining against the ulcer-causing effects of NSAIDs. It is even formulated as a combination medication with the NSAID diclofenac, which is marketed as a "stomach-safe" NSAID under the brand name Arthrotec. Misoprostol sometimes causes a pronounced laxative effect, however. Although this can be an unacceptable side effect, many cancer patients taking opioids suffer chronic constipation, which may actually make this side effect an additional benefit of the medication.

Other Side Effects

In patients who have kidney disease and a few other conditions, NSAIDs can cause a rise in the blood levels of a waste product, creatinine, that is removed by the kidneys. In rare cases, NSAIDs can even cause kidney failure. Using injections of ketorolac for more than five days has been particularly associated with kidney failure.

Kidney injury can occur with few symptoms until the patient begins to retain fluid and experiences swelling. By the time swelling becomes apparent, however, the damage has usually progressed to an advanced point. For this reason, it is important to monitor patients on chronic NSAID therapy by checking blood pressure and performing blood tests for creatinine and urea nitrogen (BUN) every three months. If the BUN or creatinine rises significantly or if hypertension develops or worsens, the NSAIDs should be discontinued. In those few cases of kidney failure caused by NSAID toxicity, the kidney damage is usually temporary. Kidney function generally returns a few weeks after the patient stops taking the drug. Some factors that put people at high risk of kidney-related side effects from NSAIDs are:

- Older than sixty
- Kidney disease (interstitial nephritis, papillary necrosis, chronic renal failure)
- Congestive heart failure
- Cirrhosis of the liver
- Taking chemotherapy drugs that impair kidney function (cis-platinum, cyclosporine)

NSAIDs also block the action of blood structures called platelets, which are important in activating the blood-clotting mechanism. Because of this action, NSAIDs can slightly increase the risk of bleeding from surgery or other invasive procedures. This can be especially significant for patients taking anticoagulant (blood-thinning) drugs such as coumadin. In certain conditions, such as following heart attacks, NSAIDs such as aspirin are specifically used to disable platelets and reduce the risk of further clotting.

NSAIDs may also increase blood pressure, especially in elderly persons. The average patient's blood pressure will rise about 10 mm after beginning an NSAID medication. NSAIDs can also interfere with the actions of some commonly used antihypertensive medications such as beta-blockers (propranolol, atenolol, metoprolol) and ACE-inhibitors (captopril, benazepril, lisinopril).

Indomethacin (Indocin), a very potent NSAID sometimes used to treat bone pain in cancer patients, tends to accumulate in the brain. This sometimes causes temporary confusion or drowsiness, especially in the elderly. A few other NSAIDs have also been reported to cause drowsiness, but this seems to be a very rare effect.

Acetaminophen (Tylenol) does not cause stomach, kidney, or platelet problems. When used in excess (more than 4,000 mg per day for a prolonged period) or in people who have liver disease (such as chronic hepatitis or alcoholism), acetaminophen can cause significant liver damage. Most people would never knowingly take such high doses, but many different over-the-counter pain medications contain some acetaminophen, as do some short-acting opioid medications. People with chronic pain often unknowingly take two or three different medications containing acetaminophen.

Specific (COX-2) NSAIDs

The prostaglandins that cause inflammation and pain are made by a different mechanism than the prostaglandins that maintain stomach, kidney, and platelet function. The pain-causing prostaglandins are produced by an enzyme called cyclooxygenase 2 (COX-2); those that are used for routine body functions are created by a slightly different enzyme, cyclooxygenase 1 (COX-1). Most NSAIDs inhibit both COX-1 and COX-2 enzymes. The inhibition of COX-2 enzymes is responsible for pain relief, while the inhibition of COX-1 enzymes is responsible for most side effects.

Some of the NSAIDs are more active against COX-1 than COX-2, and therefore are more likely to cause stomach irritation and other side effects. These include aspirin (which is over a hundred times more active against COX-1 than it is against COX-2), indomethacin (Indocin), and piroxicam (Feldene). Others, such as naproxen (Naprosyn, Anaprox) and diclofenac (Voltaren), have less anti-COX-1 effects and are associated with fewer side effects. Nabumetone (Relafen) has been shown to cause less irritation of the stomach and esophagus than the other NSAIDs.

In the past two years, a new class of medications has been developed called selective COX-2 inhibitors. The first of these medications released in the United States was celecoxib (Celebrex). It is four hundred times more active against COX-2 than COX-1, so theoretically it should have far fewer side effects than the other NSAIDs. Studies have shown that celecoxib is far less likely to cause gastric bleeding than the standard NSAIDs, although it may still cause painful stomach irritation. However, celecoxib is chemically similar to the sulfa drugs (a group of antibiotics) and has been associated with severe skin reactions in patients who are allergic to sulfa medications.

Another selective COX-2 inhibitor, refocoxib (Vioxx), has recently been introduced. Like celecoxib, it is supposed to have the pain relieving and anti-inflammatory effects of NSAIDs with fewer side effects. Early studies show the medication does have fewer side effects, but it sometimes causes kidney problems similar to those caused by the other NSAIDs.

The COX-2 inhibitors do have fewer side effects than traditional NSAIDs, but they are no more effective as pain relievers. They are also more expensive. Currently, there is little information on the use of COX-2 inhibitors in the treatment of cancer pain. Common sense would indicate they could be useful for those who get relief from NSAIDs but who are unable to tolerate the side effects. There is no reason to believe they will give pain relief to persons who have not received pain relief from other NSAIDs, however.

Guidelines for Choosing NSAIDs for Cancer Pain

The National Comprehensive Cancer Network published guidelines for the use of NSAIDs for cancer pain in 1999, before there was much experience with the selective COX-2 inhibiting medications. Since individual responses to NSAIDs are so variable, the first recommendation is that a person with mild cancer pain should use any NSAID that was effective and well tolerated in the past. If the person has not taken NSAIDs before, reasonable first choices, starting doses, and maximum doses are:

Ibuprofen (Motrin), 400 mg 4 times per day (up to 3,200 mg per day).

Fenoprofen (Nalfon), 400 mg 4 times per day (up to 3,200 mg per day).

Sulindac (Clinoril), 150 mg twice a day (up to 400 mg per day).

For patients who are at increased risk of bleeding problems, because of recent surgery, coumadin therapy, or low platelet counts from chemotherapy, the guidelines recommend the use of an NSAID that does not inhibit platelet function. These include:

Choline magnesium trisalicylate (Trilisate), 500 mg 3 times per day (up to 4,500 mg per day).

Salsalate (Disalcid, Salgesic), 500 mg twice daily (up to 3,000 mg per day).

Acetaminophen (Tylenol), 1,000 mg (2 extra strength tablets) every 6 hours.

Of course, there are dozens of NSAIDs. There is no need to try all of them, but most recommendations are to try different ones until you have found at least two that you can take without side effects. If two different NSAIDs are used without reducing the pain, NSAIDs probably will not be effective and should be discontinued. If an NSAID medication is effective but its use is limited by a side effect, try a different NSAID that is less likely to cause that side effect. Alternatively, it may be better to treat the side effect and continue NSAID therapy.

If an NSAID relieves some of the pain, but not enough to allow a return to normal function, it may still be useful when taken with an opioid (narcotic) pain reliever. In general, NSAIDs and opioid medications used in combination provide more pain relief than either medication alone. There is no convincing evidence that using two different NSAIDs (or an NSAID and acetaminophen) at the same time offers any advantage over the use of either one alone. The one possible exception may be in the case of high fevers caused by tumors, when traditional NSAIDs used in combination with acetaminophen may reduce the temperature more than either one does alone.

It is important to note that many of the currently used opioid medications already come as combinations with NSAIDs. The NSAIDs most frequently used in these combinations include aspirin (Percodan), acetaminophen (Percocet, Tylox, Tylenol #3, Vicodin, Lortab, Roxicet), and ibuprofen (Vicoprofen). Some people unknowingly continue to take their NSAID medications when they start on one of these combination medications. In that situation, it is important to consult your physician or to stop the NSAID in order to avoid taking a toxic dose.

Adjunctive Medications

The remainder of this chapter deals with adjunctive (additional or helping) medications. These medications are called adjuvant because they are used in addition to other pain-relieving medications such as NSAIDs and opioids. Many cancer patients will never need any of these medicines; their pain is well controlled with routine medications. Much of the experience with using adjuvant medications has come from the treatment of chronic pain from noncancerous causes. Although many of these medications are widely used in pain clinics, some cancer specialists are unaware of their use for treating cancer pain.

Adjuvant medications are especially important for the 10 to 20 percent of cancer patients whose pain is not relieved by opioids. Opioid-resistant pain is unusual early in the course of cancer. These medications may be needed to treat the more severe pain of advanced cancer, especially if the tumor or treatment has caused neuropathic pain (see chapters 1 and 2). When sensory nerves are damaged by cancer, surgery, chemotherapy, or radiation, they may send abnormal impulses into the central nervous system, causing the burning, shooting sensations characteristic of neuropathic pain.

Neuropathic pain can be constant or intermittent, but it almost always feels different from other types of pain. In addition to the burning sensation, words used to describe neuropathic pain often include electric, tingling, painfully numb, itching, crawling feeling, or raw. Neuropathic pain rarely improves with NSAIDs and responds only partially to opioids, even at high doses. The adjunctive medications can often improve neuropathic pain dramatically, but may take several weeks to become effective. When even adjunctive medications fail, more invasive therapies (see chapters 10 and 11) may be required.

Antidepressants

Antidepressant medications have been used to treat chronic pain for more than twenty-five years. The tricyclic antidepressants (TCA) seem to work better for this purpose than other antidepressant medications. In the United States, more than half of all the prescriptions for tricyclic antidepressant medications are given for pain rather than for depression. TCAs can stimulate the body's natural pain-relieving pathways and thus increase the analgesic effects of opioid medications. They may also increase the blood level of a given dose of some opioid medications, helping them to work even more effectively. This effect has already been demonstrated for morphine and methadone and may occur with other opioids.

Unlike NSAIDs or opioids, a TCA medication does not relieve pain an hour or two after taking it. Rather, the medication must be taken steadily for several days, after which the severity of pain gradually lessens. The pain-relieving effect usually begins anywhere from four days to three weeks after starting on the medication and taking it regularly. The dosage needed to relieve pain is generally far less than the dosage required to treat depression.

There are many different TCA medications to choose from (see Table 4.1). Amitriptyline (Elavil) may be the most potent pain reliever of the commonly used TCA medications, but it is also the most sedating. It should not be used by people with glaucoma, enlarged prostates, or cardiac arrhythmias. If amitriptyline is too sedating, nortriptyline (Pamelor) may be more useful. Imipramine (Tofranil) and doxepin (Sinequan) may also be more tolerable. Desipramine (Norpramine) has been found to be especially useful for treating neuropathic pain, and it also has less sedative effects than most other TCAs. In some patients, desipramine also acts as a mild stimulant, which may be beneficial for persons sedated from high doses of opioids. Clomipramine (Anafranil) may be one of the most potent TCAs in terms of analgesia, but its use has been limited by side effects that can include convulsions and liver toxicity.

The analgesic effects of the tricyclics are independent of their antidepressant effects. The analgesic effects occur more quickly and at lower doses. While the degree of pain relief given by TCAs is modest when compared to that of the opioids, TCAs can be given in combination with opioid medications to increase their analgesic effects. TCAs may also be more effective against certain types of pain, particularly neuropathic (nerve damage) pain with burning or shooting sensations. Although the analgesic effects of TCAs may be seen within a week of starting the medication, a reasonable trial should last from six to twelve weeks.

Some people are very sensitive to TCAs and suffer disturbing side effects, such as heavy sedation or bad dreams, even from low doses of the medication. Paradoxically, this can predict a good response, if they are able to continue. This may mean starting with a very small dose of medication at bedtime (especially for elderly people) and slowly increasing the dose as the side effects lessen (which will happen over time). Usually, the dose can be increased 25 to 50 percent every three to four days. For other people, the sedation caused by the tricyclics simply helps them sleep, sometimes resulting in their first good night's sleep in months.

The other possible side effects of the TCAs (see Table 4.3 for a list of common side effects) include morning sedation, a drop in blood pressure on standing (postural hypotension), and dry mouth. All these side effects usually disappear within two weeks on a stable dose of the medication. Some patients report weight gain due to appetite stimulation, which is often a good thing for cancer patients. A few people experience constipation. Very rarely, female patients may start lactating (producing breast milk) while taking tricyclics. This will resolve after stopping the medication. Overdoses of TCAs can cause life-threatening cardiac arrhythmias (abnormal heartbeats), which can make these drugs especially dangerous for patients who are at risk of taking an accidental or purposeful overdose.

The newer class of antidepressants, the selective serotonin reuptake inhibitors (SSRIs), have largely replaced the tricyclic medications for the treatment of depression. These medications have not been as well studied for pain-relieving effects as have the tricyclics. However, at least one of the newer SSRI antidepressants, paroxetine (Paxil), has been shown to have some pain-relieving effects of its own. There is also evidence that citalopram (Celexa) may relieve pain to a modest degree. However, another drug in this class, fluoxetine (Prozac), has no significant pain-relieving effects, though it remains an excellent antidepressant medication. It should be noted that SSRIs can reduce the effectiveness of certain opioids, particularly oxycodone and hydrocodone, which must be activated in the liver before they are effective.

The SSRIs have a more rapid effect against depression than do the TCAs. They also tend to be stimulating rather than sedating (although this effect does not occur in every individual). SSRIs are also safer if an overdose is taken. For these reasons, most doctors now prefer to use SSRIs to treat symptoms of depression in cancer patients and to use TCAs to treat pain and to improve sleep.

Some doctors like to give an SSRI in the morning and a small dose of a TCA at night. This combination can be very effective in persons with depression and pain. It should be noted, however, that the two types of medications interact, causing an increase in the blood level of the tricyclic medication. For this reason, only small doses of TCA should be used.

A few antidepressants have some characteristics of both SSRIs and TCAs. One such medication is venlafaxine (Effexor). It is not clear yet if these medications are effective as pain relievers, but there is some evidence that they are. As with the other antidepressants, however, the pain-relieving effects may not be apparent for several weeks. Venlafaxine can cause elevations in blood pressure and frequently causes nausea, which limits its use in many cases.

Anticonvulsants

Anticonvulsants are medications used to control epilepsy (seizures). Seizures are caused by damaged neurons (nerve cells) in the brain that send out abnormal signals. If the abnormal signal spreads throughout the brain, a seizure results. Anticonvulsants work by suppressing these abnormal nerve signals and preventing their spread to other neurons. It makes sense that these medications could also suppress the abnormal nerve signals that cause neuropathic pain.

Anticonvulsant medications have been used to treat neuropathic pain problems, such as the pain of shingles, for more than thirty years. They have also been used to treat the pain arising from nerves damaged by many other conditions. However, anticonvulsants have probably not been used as frequently as they should be for treating cancer pain, perhaps because cancer specialists are not very familiar with these medications. The use of anticonvulsants for pain treatment often requires several dosage adjustments over a few weeks. An oncologist who is primarily focused on treating the tumor itself may not have time to handle antiseizure medication adjustments in addition to the other treatments he must oversee. For this reason, it may be necessary to consult a neurologist or pain specialist who can prescribe the antiseizure medications.

The most commonly used anticonvulsant for the treatment of pain is gabapentin (Neurontin). It seems to be quite helpful for pain caused by nerve damage, the peripheral neuropathy that follows certain chemotherapies, and pain problems that follow radiation treatments (see chapter 3). It is especially effective in treating painful conditions that involve electrical or shooting pain sensations. It effectively reduces hypersensitivity in areas where light touch or mild temperature changes feel painful (allodynia). Overall, about half the patients with these symptoms will get significant pain relief from gabapentin. Many people with neuropathic pain find that gabapentin relieves pain more effectively than do opioids. Gabapentin also improves the quality of sleep and, in some people, has mild mood-elevating effects.

Gabapentin is not broken down by the body; it is excreted by the kidneys in its unchanged form. Because of this, it does not interact with other medications and can be safely used even by persons with severe liver disease. The side effects of gabapentin are quite variable, but the most common reported problems are dizziness, sleepiness, or swelling (which can usually be managed with diuretic medications). These side effects occur frequently, but they are usually mild and will stop after the patient has taken the medication for a week or two. In about 15 percent of people, however, the side effects are too severe for them to continue taking the medication.

A common starting dose of gabapentin is 300 mg three times per day, although much lower starting doses (100 mg three times a day) are given to elderly patients. Some physicians give the entire dose at bedtime to avoid daytime sedation. The dose of gabapentin can be increased by 300 mg per day every three to five days until there is pain relief. Some people will experience pain relief at doses as low as 300 mg per day, while others will need more than 3,000 mg per day. If no relief is obtained after several weeks at the highest tolerated dose, gabapentin should be stopped and a different antiseizure medication tried.

Although the other antiseizure medications are not used as frequently for pain treatment, they are sometimes effective when gabapentin causes side effects or does not work well. Carbamazepine (Tegretol, Epitrol) is an anticonvulsant that has been available for nearly forty years. It has long been used for a variety of neuropathic pain syndromes and to treat cancer pain caused by nerve damage. Carbamazepine may also have some anti-depressant effects. The usual dose is 200 mg once in the evening, slowly increased to 200 mg three times per day over two weeks or so. In a few cases, doses as high as 600 mg three times a day have been used.

Carbamazepine should be taken with food. Common side effects include nausea, dizziness, problems with coordination, and sedation. If these side effects occur in a patient who is getting good pain relief from the medication, a useful strategy is to discontinue the drug completely for twenty-four hours and then resume treatment, lowering the daily dose by 200 mg. The most serious side effect of carbamazepine is a decrease in the number of white blood cells (neutropenia), which can put a person at risk for serious infection. Neutropenia only occurs in a few people and usually becomes apparent during the first three months of treatment. It is important, however, that every person taking carbamazepine have her blood count checked after taking the medication for a few weeks.

Other anticonvulsants that have shown some benefit in the treatment of neuropathic pain include phenytoin (Dilantin), phenobarbital (Primidone), and valproate (Depakote), but these are generally not used to treat cancer pain. Lamotrigine (Lamictal) is a new anticonvulsant that has been effective against a few cases of neuropathic pain that did not respond to the other anticonvulsants. It has been associated with severe and even dangerous skin rashes if the dose is escalated too quickly, however, so many doctors prefer not to use it.

Benzodiazepines

The benzodiazepine class of medications includes the minor tranquilizers such as diazepam (Valium), lorazepam (Ativan), and oxazepam (Serax), as well as many of the commonly used sleeping pills. All these medications work at a chemical receptor in the brain called GABA-A. In addition to their tranquilizing effects, all the benzodiazepines cause sedation and may impair memory and thinking ability, especially when they are first started.

There is considerable controversy over using the benzodiazepine medications to treat pain. Some physicians feel that benzodiazepines are inappropriate for the treatment of chronic pain because they are habit-forming and have a high potential for abuse. Many feel that when the benzodiazepines seem to be effective, they are simply relieving anxiety.

However, several studies have found that certain benzodiazepines, such as alprazolam (Xanax), have pain-relieving effects that are unrelated to their sedative or tranquilizing effects. These medications seem particularly effective for treating muscle spasms and certain types of pain originating in the muscles. Of course, benzodiazepines are also helpful for treating anxiety and insomnia. While these symptoms may not be considered painful, they can certainly add to the discomfort that cancer patients experience.

Alprazolam may be especially effective for treating pain because it has some actions that are similar to those of the tricyclic antidepressant medications, including a direct effect on pain receptors in the central nervous system. There is some evidence that alprazolam might even have some opioidlike effects of its own, because some of the drug's effects can be neutralized by opioid-reversing medications like naloxone (Narcan). In a recent study of patients with chronic pain, 73 percent showed improvement after two weeks of low-dose alprazolam (0.5 mg three times per day). Alprazolam also appears to have a synergistic effect with opioid medications. This means that the amount of pain relief obtained when the two medications are given together is more than would be expected from simply adding the amount of pain relief each gives alone.

Although alprazolam has few side effects, persons taking it for a long time can become physically dependent on the medication and will have withdrawal symptoms if it is stopped suddenly. Unfortunately, dependence on alprazolam is more difficult to treat than dependence on the other benzodiazepines. If a person wants to stop alprazolam after taking it for several months, it is usually best to substitute another benzodiazepine for a month or more, and then slowly taper that medication.

Another benzodiazepine, clonazepam (Klonopin), has some effects similar to those of gabapentin and may be effective in treating neuropathic pain. It is generally used in doses of 0.25 to 1.0 mg given three times per day. As with other benzodiazepines, tolerance and dependence can occur, but this is unusual in patients who take the clonazepam for less than six months in low doses.

Another commonly used medicine for muscle spasm, carisoprodol (Soma), may exert its pain-relieving effects through the actions of one of its breakdown products, meprobamate, which is structurally similar to the benzodiazepines. Carisoprodol is often used as an antispasmodic (see below), but it can be a very habit-forming drug, and some patients develop a strong physical dependence on it.

Antispasmodics

Antispasmodic medications are generally used for abnormal contractions (spasms or cramps) of the muscles. Two very different groups of medications are used. One group is used only to treat spasms of the skeletal muscles, such as those in the back and legs. Other medications are used for spasms of the smooth muscles located in the visceral organs, such as the intestines, bladder, and esophagus. A few medications can be used to treat both types of muscle spasms. Most antispasmodics are not particularly effective as pain relievers, but the relief of spasms may itself reduce pain. Two of these medications, baclofen and clonidine, are frequently used for the treatment of cancer pain. A few others are used occasionally.

Baclofen (Lioresal) is a powerful antispasmodic medication that is often used to control muscle spasms caused by spinal cord injuries or multiple sclerosis. It is also useful for the treatment of severe bowel or bladder spasms. Baclofen has proven useful for the treatment of chronic neuropathic pain and may add to the effects of the antiseizure medications when used for that purpose.

Baclofen is related to the benzodiazepines, but it acts on a slightly different receptor called GABA-B. Not surprisingly, the side effects of baclofen are similar to those of the benzodiazepines and include sedation, dizziness, and sometimes confusion. At high doses, baclofen may also inhibit the release of chemicals called excitatory amino acids in the central nervous system. These chemicals are one of the brain's primary messengers for somatic and visceral pain signals. Some of baclofen's pain-relieving effects may occur by this mechanism.

Baclofen is usually started at a dose of 5 mg three times per day. It can be increased slowly up to 20 mg taken four times per day. Some people are able to tolerate even higher doses, which may be used if the benefits outweigh the side effects. The muscle relaxation effect usually begins within three to four days, but the peak effect of this medication usually is not apparent until about ten days after starting on a particular dose.

Baclofen may relieve pain by its effects in both the spinal cord and the brain. It is particularly useful for patients who suffer bowel or bladder spasms after undergoing radiation treatment to the abdomen or pelvis. Baclofen has also proven to be effective in neuropathic pain syndromes that do not respond well to anticonvulsants.

Another antispasmodic medication, tiazidine (Zanaflex), holds promise as a pain-relieving medication. Tiazidine acts on an entirely different receptor in the central nervous system than do the benzodiazepines and baclofen, the alpha-2 receptor. This receptor appears to be an important part of the body's natural pain-relieving system.

Tiazidine's effects begin within an hour of taking the medication and last for about six hours after each dose. The side effects, sedation and dry mouth, are usually not severe and can be minimized by increasing the dose of the drug slowly. The usual starting dose of tiazidine is 4 mg at bedtime. This is gradually increased to a dose of 4 to 8 mg taken three times per day. Tiazidine's effects may be additive to those of baclofen, and the two medications may be used together in cases of severe spasms.

Another medication that acts on the alpha-2 receptor is clonidine (Catapres), which was originally developed as an antihypertensive (high blood pressure) medication. Clonidine is a very effective pain reliever, but its use as a pain medication is limited by its effects on blood pressure. Most persons who take clonidine by mouth will begin to suffer symptoms of low blood pressure long before they obtain significant pain relief. However, clonidine has become a very useful pain medication when administered directly into the cerebrospinal fluid via an intrathecal pump (see chapter 11).

There are other medications that are often used to treat skeletal muscle spasm, including cyclobenzaprine (Flexeril), methocarbamol (Robaxin), and orphendrine (Norgesic). The major effect of these medications is mild sedation. They do not appear to be useful in relieving pain, and there is considerable doubt as to whether they actually cause any muscle relaxation.

Antiarrhythmics

Antiarrhythmic medications are used to treat irregular heartbeats. Many of these medications are similar chemically to local anesthetics. Some studies hint these medications may be helpful in treating neuropathic pain. Mexiletine (Mexitil) is the antiarrhythmic medication most often used for this purpose, and it sometimes benefits the pain of peripheral neuropathy, radiation-induced pelvic pain, and other neuropathic pains. It is usually considered a drug of last resort, however, used only for patients who have not responded to other treatments.

No one is certain why mexiletine may be pain relieving. It stabilizes nerve cell membranes, so perhaps it keeps damaged nerves from sending out abnormal pain messages. It also inhibits the release of substance P, a pain-transmitting chemical, in the central nervous system. Mexiletine can be started at a dose of 150 mg at bedtime, which is then increased to three times per day (taken with food) as tolerated. It usually requires taking a dose of 150 mg three times per day for more than two weeks before pain relief is obtained.

Mexiletine is associated with frequent side effects; the most common are hypotension (low blood pressure) and nausea. Almost half the patients who try mexiletine will stop the medication because of these effects. Additionally, because the drug has effects on the heart, an electrocardiogram must be performed before starting the medication and after taking it for several days. Certain cardiac conditions, particularly certain types of "heart block," are contraindications to taking mexiletine. Patients who have a history of seizures should also avoid this drug.

Because mexiletine is occasionally very effective, but frequently causes side effects, doctors have searched for a way to predict which patients will benefit from the drug. One controversial study has suggested that the effectiveness of mexiletine can be predicted by giving lidocaine (another local anesthetic and antiarrhythmic drug) intravenously. Some patients obtain good pain relief for hours or days following the lidocaine injection, while others experience no relief. It has been suggested (again controversially) that only those patients who obtain relief from lidocaine are likely to benefit from mexiletine.

Stimulants

Stimulants such as amphetamine (Dexedrine) and methylphenidate (Ritalin) have found limited use as adjuvant medications for treating cancer pain. Their primary use is to counteract the sedation in patients who require high doses of opioid medications. In some cases, they may actually augment the pain-relief effects of opioids. Doses of 5 to 10 mg (usually given in the morning and again at noon) have been very effective in enhancing the comfort of terminally ill cancer patients. They may be especially useful for geriatric patients in whom the medications increase activity levels while decreasing pain and sedation.

The side effects of stimulants include anxiety, tremulousness, loss of appetite, and, rarely, psychological effects, including delirium (severe mental disturbance, sometimes including hallucinations) or paranoia. Methylphenidate, which has a shorter duration of action than the other stimulants, is usually better tolerated.

Corticosteroids (Steroids or Cortisone)

Corticosteroids have proven very effective, especially for the short-term (less than four weeks) treatment of bone pain, pain due to nerve compression, pain from partial bowel obstruction, and headaches due to brain tumors. Corticosteroids are also effective as appetite stimulants. Most of these medications, particularly dexamethasone (Decadron, Hexadrol), have some mood-elevating effects, but these effects rarely last more than a month, even with continuous daily use. For mild to moderate pain requiring steroids, prednisone (Deltasone) or methylprednisolone (Medrol) are frequently used. The most effective steroid for the pain of nerve compression is dexamethasone.

Common side effects of corticosteroids include fluid retention, appetite stimulation, gastritis (NSAIDs should not be used at the same time as steroids), and high blood pressure. Corticosteroids also cause elevated blood sugar and therefore should be used with extreme caution by people with diabetes. With chronic use (every day for more than a month), steroids can cause susceptibility to serious infections, muscle weakness, and osteoporosis.

Some people become excitable or anxious while taking steroids, and the medications may cause insomnia. For this reason, these medications are generally administered as a single daily dose in the morning. A few people develop significant psychiatric side effects, ranging from irritability to delusions and psychosis.

Rarely Used Medications

Cannabinoids

There has been a lot of attention paid in the popular press lately to the use of cannabinoid drugs—specifically marijuana—for the treatment of pain and other symptoms of cancer. The major active ingredient in marijuana, delta-9-tetrahydrocannabinol (THC), is currently available by doctor's prescription in all states in a capsule form called dronabinol (Marinol). Some states have even legalized the use of herbal marijuana for the treatment of cancer pain.

Although there are many individual testimonials about the effectiveness of marijuana, there have not been extensive studies of the use of cannabinoids for treating cancer pain. Doses of dronabinol of 15 to 20 mg have been shown to produce significant pain relief in a small study of patients with cancer pain. At this dose, however, most of the patients also reported psychiatric side effects such as depersonalization, anxiety, or disconnected thoughts. In another study, 10 mg of dronabinol was found to give the same amount of pain relief as 60 mg of codeine (a weak opioid), but the side effects of dronabinol were more pronounced. One indication that dronabinol has not been very effective is the small number of prescriptions written for it in the United States since it came on the market.

Advocates of smoking marijuana instead of taking dronabinol point out that the herb contains more than four hundred other chemicals that may have analgesic effects not found in the purified dronabinol. Opponents of marijuana counter that it also contains chemicals that can cause psychosis and that smoking an impure plant, which may contain fungal particles and pesticides, is an especially hazardous way to deliver medications to cancer patients. At this time, however, there are no studies that clearly show if the pain-relieving effects of smoking marijuana are (or are not) superior to those of dronabinol.

There are fairly convincing studies, however, that dronabinol is effective in treating the nausea and vomiting associated with cancer chemotherapy. Dronabinol does not seem to be any more effective than other medications available for that purpose, but it is certainly possible that it works better in some individuals. A few studies also indicate that dronabinol may increase appetite, and the National Institute of Health does recognize the effectiveness of dronabinol for increasing appetite in cancer patients. Again, however, there are several other drugs at least as effective for the same purpose.

NMDA-Receptor Inhibitors

The chemicals that carry the signal for chronic pain work by stimulating nerve cells in the spinal cord and the brain. In addition to the opioid receptor, these cells also contain another receptor called the NMDA receptor. When enough pain signals have been generated for a prolonged period of time, the nerve cells start to expose more of these NMDA receptors on their surfaces. Stimulation of these receptors is associated with worsening pain, hypersensitivity to pain, and the development of tolerance (loss of effect at the same dose) to opioid medications. These receptors can be blocked by drugs called, appropriately enough, NMDA-receptor inhibitors. One such medication is ketamine (Ketocet), which is generally used as an anesthetic agent.

Small amounts of ketamine, in doses below those used for anesthesia, can make the opioid medications work more effectively, particularly in patients who have had pain for a long time. Ketamine can be given orally, by injection, or as a nasal spray. In higher doses, ketamine can cause psychosis, so its use for pain treatment must be limited. It may be useful, however, for terminal patients whose pain cannot be relieved by other means.

Other medications that can act as NMDA-receptor inhibitors are amantidine (which is generally used to treat Parkinson's disease and viral infections) and dextromethorphan (which is available in over-the-counter cough syrups). Methadone, a long-acting opioid, also has NMDA-receptor inhibitor activity. This may be a reason why methadone is sometimes effective against cancer pain that is not relieved by other opioids.

Capsaicin

Capsaicin (pronounced "cap-say-sin") is a substance that is extracted from red chili peppers. The heat that these peppers cause on the tongue is actually a brief episode of neuropathic pain. The sensation occurs because a chemical in the peppers causes the release of the neurotransmitter substance P from nerve endings in the tongue.

It is commonly known that people who eat chili peppers regularly do not suffer as much from the peppers' effects as do people who eat them rarely. This is because regular use of the peppers actually depletes the stores of substance P in the nerve fibers of the tongue. Once these fibers have run out of substance P, they cannot generate pain signals.

In 1940, a Hungarian scientist realized that this effect of hot peppers might be useful for pain treatment. He isolated the active ingredient capsaicin and formulated it into a cream. Capsaicin cream is currently available over-the-counter as Zostrix cream. It is sometimes effective for neuropathic pain involving the skin or joints. The cream must be applied routinely (two or three times per day) for two to three weeks before it works.

People who use capsaicin must be aware that after the first application they will often feel a burning sensation and tenderness at the site that may last for twenty-four to forty-eight hours. Their pain may actually increase for the first week or two. After multiple applications, however, capsaicin will no longer cause any sensitivity in the area where it is applied. Soon afterward, most patients report that their chronic burning pain has lessened. Capsaicin has proven particularly useful for postmastectomy pain syndrome.

Other Drugs That Enhance the Effects of Opioids

Several medications may help the opioid medications to work more effectively. In general, the effects of these medications are small, but in some cases they may make the difference between effective pain relief and inadequate pain relief.

Hydroxyzine (Atarax, Vistaril) is an antihistamine that enhances the analgesic effects of opioids and has some analgesic effects of its own. Other than sedation, it has few side effects. Because of its sedative effect, hydroxyzine is often used as a bedtime medication.

Propranolol (Inderal) has occasionally helped relieve the pain of central pain syndromes that sometimes occur after a stroke, after the removal of brain tumors from certain areas, or following irradiation of the brain. Propranolol may also help opioid medications work more effectively. There is also evidence that some of the calcium channel blocking medications (usually used for hypertension) can also enhance the effects of opioid medications. All these medications can have significant effects on blood pressure and heart function, however, and should only be prescribed by a doctor who is quite familiar with your overall medical condition.

CHAPTER 7

Alternative Ways of Delivering Medications

by Roger S. Cicala, M.D.

W hen most people think about medicine, they consider it to be a pill or liquid taken by mouth. Most cancer patients and others who have been seriously ill might think about receiving medication by injection or through an intravenous catheter (IV) while in the hospital. For most people, these are the only ways they will ever take pain medicines, or any other medicine for that matter.

Most people never consider that there might be a need to take medications in another way. However, there are many cases when, for a number of reasons, oral medications do not work well. Injected pain medication can provide good relief when this happens, but taking four or five shots a day is not always possible, or pleasant. Giving the medications by a continuous intravenous drip may be an alternative that is appropriate and effective for people who are bedridden or housebound. For those who are more active, however, continuous IV infusion means always being attached to an infusion pump, something that is limiting at best. It is also quite expensive. For example, a pain medication that costs about $6 a day by mouth costs about $170 a day by intravenous infusion.

A variety of options are available for patients who need medications delivered in other ways. Some of the alternatives are as high tech as implanting refillable pumps to deliver medications directly into the fluid around the spinal cord and brain (see chapter 11). Most of the alternative methods discussed in this chapter are not very complicated, however, and can provide good pain relief for many people who cannot take oral medications.

Why Oral Medications May Not Work

Almost every type of pain medication (with a few important exceptions we will discuss later) is available in tablets or liquids to be taken by mouth. Any medication taken by mouth is first absorbed through the intestines and then passed to the liver, which breaks down some of the medication before it reaches the rest of the body. For this reason, the dose of pain medicine needed if taken by mouth is usually much higher than the dose needed if taken by injection (see Table 5.1 for examples). As long as a proper dose is given, however, oral medications usually work almost as well as injected medications. Oral medications do take longer to take effect, though, since they must be absorbed through the intestines before reaching the rest of the body.

When pain pills do not seem to be working, the most common cause is that the medicine just is not strong enough, or is not being given in a high enough dose. Everyone's body is a bit different, so a "usual" dose of medicine is not always efficient. The first step in correcting the problem is to try a different medication or to increase the dose. When several different oral pain medications are not effective, however, your doctor should consider that you might have a problem with oral medications.

Absorption Difficulties

We usually think that anything we take by mouth just dissolves inside and gets absorbed into our bodies, sort of the way sugar dissolves in water. In reality, the process is a lot more complicated than that. Most medications dissolve in the stomach, but are not actually absorbed until they get to the intestines. If something delays the stomach from emptying its contents into the intestines, the medicine may not have any effect for quite a long time.

People who have diabetes, for example, often have slow emptying of their stomach contents (medically, this is called gastroporesis, pronounced "gas-trow-pore-ees-iss"). When a person is nauseous, his stomach is probably not emptying well, if at all. Of course, when someone is vomiting, there is a good chance the medication will never even get to his intestines.

If the medication does get to the intestines, the actual absorption is still a pretty complicated process. The molecule of medication must pass through one of the cells lining the intestines, then through another membrane, through the lining cell of a capillary (a very small blood vessel), and finally into the bloodstream. If the medicine binds to other chemicals in the intestines, it may never get a chance to be absorbed. Antacids, for example, are notorious for binding medications this way. You probably should not take any kind of medicine for an hour before or an hour after you take an antacid. (Medications that stop acid secretion, like Tagamet or Zantac, are not a problem, but chewable or liquid antacids are.)

If the lining of the intestines is damaged, it may not be able to absorb medications (or anything else, for that matter) well. Radiation to the abdomen, recent chemotherapy, and even some viral infections can all damage the lining of the intestines. Many cancer patients have trouble absorbing medications for a few days or even a week or two after certain types of chemotherapy. Absorption problems probably affect controlled-release pills, like OxyContin or MS-Contin, more than regular, short-acting pain pills.

Absorption problems often begin subtly in cancer patients. The pain medications still work to some degree, but they begin to take longer to have an effect or don't provide as much pain relief. At first, it can be impossible to tell if this is an absorption problem, since the same thing can happen as your body gets used to taking pain medications. Over time, however, as the dose of medicine is continually increased but provides less relief, your doctor should consider that you might not be absorbing it properly.

Sometimes, absorption problems are obvious, as when a person notices she is passing intact pills in her stool, or that she vomits up an intact pill hours after taking a medication. A few time-release pills, however, are supposed to pass in the stool. These pills release their active medicine in the intestines, but the matrix (or shell) of the pill is not absorbed.

If there is a question about absorption, the simplest solution is to try an injection of the same pain medication being taken by mouth. Someone who is taking very high doses of oral medication without relief, but who gets relief with an injection of a small amount of the same medication, is probably having absorption problems. If this is the case, a different way of taking the medicine will probably be effective.

Side Effects

Some oral medications work well, but cause such severe side effects that they are almost not worth the pain relief. Most pain medications can cause nausea, at least in some people. In most cases, changing to a different type of pain medication or adding an antinausea medication will eliminate the problem or at least reduce it to an acceptable level.

All pain medications can also cause constipation. Constipation can usually be treated with milk of magnesia, fiber supplements, stool softeners, or enemas. (It is important *not* to use irritant laxatives, such as Ex-Lax or Dulcolax, however. These medications may help relieve the constipation for a time, but when used regularly will actually make the constipation worse.)

In some people, however, the nausea or constipation from oral medications is so severe that an alternative method of giving pain medicine must be tried. Some people with liver problems cannot take oral medications because their livers cannot metabolize the drug properly. This is unusual, however, since the liver has huge reserves and usually can continue to function normally even if a large portion of its tissue is damaged.

Noninvasive Methods of Delivery

There are many ways of administering pain medications besides simply taking them by mouth or giving injections. For many cancer patients, some of these alternatives can actually provide better relief than the usual methods. For others, alternative ways of taking medications allow them a lifestyle that is less limited than when they needed to take injections or pills many times each day. Most pain specialists feel that these alternative methods of giving pain medication should be used far more often than they are. In the last year or two, however, there has finally been an increase in the number of doctors who regularly prescribe them.

Unfortunately, some of the medications involved are quite expensive. Many of the companies that manufacture them, however, have "compassionate" programs to give the medications at reduced cost to cancer patients who otherwise could not afford them. Some of these companies are listed in the appendixes to this book, but your doctor can probably give you the name of the local representative in your area.

Liquids and Suppositories

The simplest alternatives to tablets and pills have been available for decades. They are not used very often, probably because they have simply been forgotten in all the hype about new medicines. Almost every type of pain medication is available in a liquid form. Liquids sometimes have advantages over pills. Because they are already in liquid form, the medication does not have to dissolve in the stomach and therefore may be absorbed into the body more quickly. Liquids can also be taken by people who have difficulty swallowing pills, or who have to be fed by tubes.

Most people do not like the thought of taking suppositories regularly, but they can have some real advantages over other methods of giving pain medicine. Because the blood supply of the rectum does not pass through the liver, medications given by suppository can get directly into the bloodstream without being metabolized the way oral medication is. Suppositories are also absorbed more quickly than oral medication, and they are absorbed even if the stomach does not empty well. They probably cause less nausea and constipation than oral medications, too.

The major disadvantage of liquids and suppositories are that no time-release or extended duration medications are available in these forms. Therefore, most suppositories only provide relief for three to five hours per dose. They are ideal, though, to use as breakthrough medications in addition to a long-acting form of pain medicine. Because generic drugs are used in suppositories and liquids, they are often less expensive than other types of pain medications.

Skin Patches

Transdermal (meaning across the skin) patches for pain control have been available for several years. The currently available patch contains the opioid medication fentanyl. This is a very potent medication that was originally developed for use in general anesthesia, providing pain control during surgery. The patches are available in several strengths under the brand name Duragesic.

Fentanyl patches have several advantages. Each patch continually releases medication for about three days, providing continuous pain relief during that time. Since the medication is absorbed directly into the bloodstream, problems with absorption from the stomach are avoided. The patches also seem to cause less constipation than oral pain medications. Nausea can still be a problem, however.

The major disadvantage of patches is that they constantly deliver the same amount of medication, whether you need it or not. For this reason, they are usually used to provide a baseline of pain relief and another medication is given for breakthrough or booster doses. Breakthrough medication is usually some type of short-acting medication.

Absorption through the skin into the bloodstream is much slower than absorption from the stomach. It may take six to eight hours after a patch is applied before it delivers an adequate dose of pain medication. The first patch may not provide peak relief for twenty-four hours. The medication remains in the skin for several hours after a patch is removed. This means that when the patches are changed, the medication from the old patch continues to work until medication from the new patch reaches the body. It also means that if a person has a side effect from patch medication, it will not clear until several hours after removal of the patch.

Gels

Some special creams and gels can pass directly through the skin and into the body. Any medications dissolved in the gel also enter the body. A number of different medications can be dissolved in these gels and used for pain control. They are usually used for localized pain, such as can occur when a tumor in one part of the body causes swelling and pain.

In general, medications given this way are most effective when the painful structures are located near the surface of the body. Nerve damage from radiation or surgery, bone pain in areas that are not covered by layers of muscle and other tissues, and pain around the head and neck may respond well to medications given in gels. In most cases, anti-inflammatory medication, or medicines that act directly on nerves, such as local anesthetics, are combined in the gels.

The medications used this way are absorbed into the bloodstream to some extent. Some doctors have tried including opioid medications in the gels for this reason. Although this does seem to work well in a few cases, it is difficult to regulate the dosage of medication given this way. For this reason, and because so many other options are available, using gels to deliver systemic (for the entire body) medications is not done very often.

Nasal Sprays

Giving medication in a nasal spray form has several advantages. The blood supply of the nasal lining does not pass through the liver, so medication absorbed here reaches the body without being metabolized by the liver. Since the membranes of the nose have a rich blood supply, the medication reaches the bloodstream almost as quickly as an injection and much more rapidly than medication taken by mouth.

The most commonly prescribed nasal spray pain medication is butorphanol (Stadol), which is available as a prepackaged medication. Other medications can be prepared in a nasal spray form, but currently these must be compounded (made from scratch) by a pharmacist. Some pharmacists are hesitant to prepare such solutions because the drugs are not approved for nasal administration.

Butorphanol nasal spray can be very effective, especially for persons who experience sudden, brief episodes of severe pain. It may also be used as a breakthrough medication in addition to other pain medications. Butorphanol is usually not appropriate for people taking very high doses of narcotic medications, however, because it may counteract the effects of the other medications to some degree. Some people also become very sedated from butorphanol, and a few people have unpleasant nightmares or suffer depression when taking it.

Lollipops, Lozenges, and Sublingual Tablets

Pain medication can also be given by methods that allow it to dissolve in the mouth, where it can be absorbed by the blood vessels in the mouth and tongue. As with nasal sprays, this method prevents the medication from going through the liver and avoids any problems with absorption from the stomach. The onset of pain relief is usually a bit slower than with a nasal spray, but much quicker than taking a pill or liquid.

It is important when using any of these types of medications that the medication remains in the mouth to be absorbed. The dosage is designed to avoid liver metabolism of the drug that would occur if it were absorbed from the stomach. If the medication is swallowed, there will not be enough to give pain relief. For this reason, you should never eat or drink anything for a few minutes after finishing the medication.

There are several varieties of manufactured lollipops containing fentanyl, the same medication used in transdermal patches. They are designed to *not* look like children's lollipops, but even so, take care to keep them (and all other medications, for that matter) away from children. Fentanyl lollipops are especially useful for people who get good relief from the patches, but need a medication for breakthrough pain. They can be used just as effectively with other types of long-acting pain medications, however.

Several other types of pain medication can be made in lozenges designed to dissolve in the mouth or tablets that can be placed under the tongue. Most of these will have to be prepared specially by a compounding pharmacist, but several manufacturers plan to release lozenges in the near future. These lozenges may (or may not, depending on the medication used) be much cheaper than the lozenges prepared by a pharmacist.

There are few problems with any of the lollipops or lozenges, other than the side effects of the medication itself, which can occur no matter how it is given. Persons who have had radiation to the mouth or throat may not absorb the medications very well, however. A few other people do not seem to get a very good effect from orally dissolved medications, for reasons that are not well understood. Infection in the mouth, such as thrush (a yeast infection), which some people develop after chemotherapy, can interfere with medication absorption.

Iontophoresis

Iontophoresis (pronounced "eye-on-toe-fore-ees-iss") means drawing a chemical across the skin by using a low-voltage electrical current. Since the molecules in most medications have an electrical charge, a direct-voltage electrical current can force them through the skin and into the bloodstream. Usually the patient does not feel the current at all, or at most feels a mild tingling sensation.

Iontophoresis is not necessary to get most medications through the skin; patches or gels can do that. It can help them get through the skin faster than they would otherwise, however. Some devices currently being tested combine both a patch and an iontophoresis device in one unit. The patch continuously releases the medication, but if the patient needs a boost, he can press a button that will administer an extra dose by iontophoresis. This can eliminate the need for a separate breakthrough medication. Such combination devices should be available by early 2001.

Alternative Methods for Administering Injectable Medications

For some cancer patients, the only way to get effective relief is through injection. This may occur near the end of the disease, when they have taken pain medications for a very long time. For others, it may be after a difficult surgery, for certain periods after chemotherapy or radiation treatments, or simply because they cannot use any of the alternative methods discussed earlier in this chapter.

For many patients in this situation, the simplest answer is simply to use a portable pump that intravenously delivers a set amount of medication each hour. In most cases, the pump is a patient-controlled analgesia (PCA) device. These devices give a steady infusion of medication and also allow the patient to push a button for an additional dose whenever he needs it. PCA devices are available for use in hospitals and at home. Most home health agencies can provide the supplies and medications to let patients use the device at home. There are also portable versions of PCA pumps that run on batteries and can be clipped to a belt or worn on a shoulder strap. These portable devices allow people to be mobile and active, no matter what kind of medication requirements they have.

In most cases, the difficulty is not with the pump or obtaining the medication, but rather with providing an intravenous (IV) line for long periods of time. The usual IV in a vein of the hand or arm has to be replaced every few days and always presents a risk of infection. For patients who need an IV for months, it is only a matter of time until all their veins have been used and it becomes difficult to start each new IV. There are several alternatives that should be considered anytime a patient requires long-term IV therapy.

Long-Term Intravenous Catheters

Many cancer patients have a permanent IV inserted when they receive chemotherapy. This may be a device such as a Port-o-cath, which is inserted surgically into one of the large veins under the collarbone and has an injection port just under the skin. These ports can sometimes be used for administering pain medications, but using them continuously increases the risk that they will become infected. Infection in a permanently implanted catheter can lead to a host of complications. It also usually means the catheter has to be removed. For this reason, some oncologists do not want pain medication given through the implanted catheter.

An alternative to surgically implanted catheters are PIC (which stands for percutaneous intravenous catheter) lines. PIC lines are long, flexible tubes inserted into a large vein, usually near the elbow. The tube (medically, all tubes are called catheters) is threaded up the vein until its tip reaches the large veins inside the chest. PIC lines do not usually require surgery for placement, so doctors may be less worried about them becoming infected. Each PIC line can remain in place for several weeks or more, so they are often used for patients who need to receive medications at home for a long time.

Neither PIC lines nor Port-o-caths are uncomfortable. Most people have no trouble being quite active with them in place. PIC lines have medical dressings over the insertion site that have to be changed every day or two and may interfere a bit with bathing, however.

Either type of catheter can be used for intermittent injections, although it is more common to use a PCA pump to deliver medication continuously, especially during the last stages of a terminal patient's disease. Most family members can quickly learn how to change the dressings and refill the medications in the pump, but home health nurses are also available to help with these tasks.

Subcutaneous Catheters

Subcutaneous catheters look exactly like IV catheters, although they may be a bit longer (three to six inches) and have a soft rubber injectable cap, rather than an opening for connecting a tube. Instead of entering a vein, the tip simply rests in the fatty tissue underneath the skin. Medication given through a subcutaneous catheter is absorbed into the body a little more slowly than it would be from an injection in the muscles.

Subcutaneous catheters are not used very frequently anymore, largely because we now have better methods of gaining access into veins, such as PIC lines. They can still be useful in a few cases, however. Some people, for example, only need an injection of medication once in a while, but do not have a family member who is comfortable learning how to give a shot. In such cases, the medication can be injected through the soft rubber cap of the subcutaneous catheter, which almost anyone can learn to do in a few seconds. The catheters can also be used in people for whom inserting a PIC line is inappropriate, such as a person who only needs injectable pain medications for a few days after a chemotherapy treatment.

The catheters are cared for in the same way as an IV site. They are covered with a small dressing that is changed every day or two. The catheter itself can stay in place for about a week without being changed. Changing the catheter is as simple as starting a new IV. A home health nurse or even a family member can insert a new catheter in a few seconds. Unfortunately, constant infusion of pain medication through a subcutaneous catheter usually does not work well.

CHAPTER 8

Palliative Treatment for Pain Control

*by Daniel Brookoff, M.D., and
Roger S. Cicala, M.D.*

P alliative means providing relief without curing. Technically, all the other therapies discussed in this book are palliative, since their focus is to treat uncomfortable symptoms without trying to cure the disease. When discussing cancer, however, palliative usually refers to using treatments that are sometimes curative, such as radiation or chemotherapy, to provide symptom relief without trying to cure the disease. For example, a surgeon may open a patient's abdomen to find an incurable tumor nearly obstructing the intestines. He may perform a palliative operation to reroute the intestines around the tumor, relieving the obstruction.

Chemotherapy, and to a lesser extent radiation therapy, are sometimes prescribed for patients with incurable cancer to extend their life expectancies. They may also be used later in the course of the cancer to provide pain relief. Palliative therapy is often used to shrink large tumors that are causing pain by pressing on other structures, or to relieve pain from tumors eroding into bone.

Palliative radiation therapy is used for pain control more often than chemotherapy is, for several reasons. Radiation therapy is often more acceptable to the patient, who may have had unpleasant experiences with chemotherapy. It can also be used to treat only specific areas, such as pain arising from a single metastatic tumor in a bone. Radiation may also have fewer adverse effects on the body than chemotherapy, which can be very important for a chronically ill patient.

Chemotherapy is used for palliative treatment in certain situations, particularly when several different tumors are causing pain in several different areas. Recently, chemotherapy has also been used for general pain control, with impressive success. It is important to realize that when chemotherapy is used in this manner, lower doses are required than were used during attempts to cure the cancer. For this reason, there are usually far fewer side effects, and those that do occur are much less severe.

Palliative Radiation Therapy

For more than one hundred years, physicians have used radiation therapy to shrink tumors and destroy cancer cells. Radiation remains one of the most effective cancer treatments when the cancer is localized to specific areas of the body, especially when those areas contain types of tissue that are tolerant to radiation.

Even in cases when a cancer is no longer curable, radiation treatments can slow cancer growth and shrink tumors. Of course, this can extend survival, but it can also relieve pain in several ways. Large tumors can cause pain by stretching or compressing surrounding tissues. Shrinking a large tumor can relieve much of this pain. Similarly, more invasive tumors grow into normal tissue causing irritation, swelling, and the destruction of the normal cells and supporting tissue (such as bone matrix), all of which cause pain. Radiation can slow cancer growth in such areas, sometimes relieving the pain in a matter of days.

Methods of Delivering Palliative Radiation

The amount of radiation that can be administered to any part of the body is limited by the effects of the radiation on the healthy tissue around the cancer. Some tissues that are generally resistant to radiation damage, such as bone, can withstand very high doses of radiation. Other areas of the body, such as the liver or intestines, cannot tolerate high doses of radiation, so treatments in these areas must be limited. The tissues most sensitive to radiation are the blood-forming cells within the bone marrow. Since these cells are present in bones throughout the body, destroying the marrow cells in one or two bones does not cause any major problems. Giving high-dose radiation to the whole body is not possible, however, unless the person is prepared to undergo a subsequent bone marrow transplant.

It's obvious, then, that the goal of radiation therapy is always to irradiate the tumor as much as possible while minimizing the amount of radiation to normal tissues. There has been great progress during the last decade in the precision with which the radiation energy can be aimed or focused, giving higher doses of radiation to the cancer cells while sparing the surrounding tissue.

External radiation is delivered as a beam from an external radiation source, usually a linear accelerator or X-ray machine. One of the newest ways of targeting a radiation beam at cancer tissue is a gamma knife. This machine targets the cancer (usually a brain tumor) with thousands of radiation beams aimed from many different angles. In this way, the cancer cells get the full impact of all the beams while individual areas of normal tissue are exposed to only a tiny fraction of the radiation energy.

Internal radiation delivers radiation to cancer cells by temporarily inserting radioactive material into a body cavity or an organ. This can be done by surgically implanting seeds of radioactive material, such as cesium-137 or iridium-192, directly into the area to receive radiation. The dose can be even more precisely regulated by surgically placing hollow tubes or catheters into the area and then loading the tubes with similar radioactive seeds. The tubes and radioactive seeds are removed after a precisely calculated dose of radiation has been given.

Some radioactive substances can also be injected into the bloodstream or taken by mouth. In these cases, the substance used is one that is selectively taken up by tissue that is the target of treatment. Orally ingested iodine-131, for example, is selectively taken up by the thyroid gland and by metastatic thyroid tumors. The rest of the body gets very little exposure from the radioactive iodine. Strontium-89, another radioactive chemical, is selectively taken up by bone tissue, so it can be used to destroy metastatic cancer invading the bones. This can be especially effective in patients who suffer pain from metastatic tumors involving several different bones.

Radiation Treatments

The effects of radiation on each different type of normal tissue are well known. The physician administering radiation therapy (a radiation oncologist) will carefully calculate the total amount of radiation that each area of the body receives. Once the safe limit has been reached in an area, no additional radiation can be given in that area without causing significant damage to the normal tissue. This is true even if the last radiation treatments were delivered years ago. In some situations, particularly when a person is suffering severe pain from tumor invasion at a site that has already received maximum radiation, the radiation oncologist may give radiation beyond the usually accepted limit.

Because normal cells heal much faster than cancer cells, dividing the radiation into a series of small treatments instead of one large treatment allows the normal tissue to recover between each session. Radiation burns and other side effects can be avoided, or at least minimized, without compromising the tumor-destroying effects of the radiation.

When a person is first evaluated for radiation treatment, the radiation oncologist will perform an examination and may obtain an X ray or CAT scan image of the area to be treated. Using this information and knowing the type of tumor involved, he can develop a detailed plan and schedule of treatment.

The next visit will involve adjusting and targeting the radiation machines and fitting lead shields around the patient to protect normal tissue from the radiation beam. The radiation therapist will take measurements and feed these readings into a computer that "remembers" the physical features of the area involved and aims the radiation beams correctly. A simulated radiation therapy session is often conducted to make sure that all the measurements are correct. This visit can take an hour to an hour and a half.

Once the simulation visit is completed, subsequent radiation treatments often take only fifteen or twenty minutes each, of which only a minute or less involves actual radiation exposure. Many patients are able to stop in for their radiation treatments on the way to work or other activities.

Implanting radioactive seeds directly into the tumor is done under general anesthesia and usually requires a surgical incision. When catheters that will be filled with radioactive material are implanted, the procedure is somewhat different. Implanting radiation catheters always involves a surgical procedure performed under general anesthesia. When you wake up, the catheters will be covered with a dressing. The radioactive material may have been placed into the catheters during surgery, but usually will be inserted a day or two after surgery. Inserting the radioactive material into the catheters is entirely painless.

The radioactive seeds are left in the catheters for five to seven days. During this time, you will be under radiation precautions. The actual amount of radiation used is small, but there are very strict government regulations that must be followed to limit the possible exposure of other people. Pregnant women and children younger than eighteen will not be allowed to visit you while the radioactive seeds are in place. Every day or two, a radiation safety officer will measure the amount of radiation being given off to make sure there is no danger to others. You may be asked to use disposable utensils when you eat, or you may have a lead-lined shield placed around your bed.

Although the precautions seem intimidating, there is actually not a great deal of radiation involved. The main purpose of the precautions is to protect health care workers who are exposed to patients with radiation implants day after day for many years. Once the seeds and catheters have been removed, your body does not remain radioactive, and you will not give off any other radiation. After that time, nothing you touch or otherwise come in contact with will be contaminated with radioactivity.

Palliative Radiation for Bone Pain

The single most common use of palliative radiation therapy is for the treatment of pain caused by tumors invading the bone. Radiation is most likely to be helpful when the primary cancer is known to be radiation sensitive. Cancers of the breast, lung, colon, skin, kidney, and gynecologic organs are usually radiation sensitive. Fortunately, these are also the types of tumors most likely to invade bones.

When a single bone is involved, external beams of radiation are usually used to destroy the tumor. Because normal bone is quite resistant to radiation damage and side effects, the entire dose of palliative radiation for bone pain can often be delivered in one treatment. When multiple areas of bone are invaded by tumor, the injection of the bone-seeking radioactive chemical strontium-89 may be used. In a few cases, radiation oncologists combine both external radiation and strontium.

In cases of very widespread, painful bone involvement, such as may occur with multiple myeloma or widespread prostatic cancer, a form of whole-body radiation can be given in two doses separated by a week or two. Each dose irradiates one-half of the body. The gap between treatments allows blood-forming cells from the unradiated side of the body to migrate and repopulate marrow cavities in the previously radiated half of the body.

Radiation treatment for tumor invading bones gives significant pain relief in 70 to 80 percent of cases, with few side effects. Pain relief is often dramatic, in some cases beginning within twenty-four hours of the first treatment. Interestingly, radiation treatment may yield significant pain relief even when the tumor does not shrink significantly.

Emergency Indications for Palliative Radiation

Two indications for palliative radiation are considered medical emergencies: tumor involving the spine and tumor causing swelling within the brain. The spread of cancer to the spine is a concern anytime a cancer patient develops a new back pain. If not treated, spinal tumors could cause compression of the spinal cord, resulting in irreversible nerve damage and paralysis.

New shooting pains, weakness in the legs, or disturbance of bowel or bladder function may all be indicators of tumors involving the spine. In such cases, an MRI scan or other test is performed to see if there is any tumor within the bones of the spine. If a spinal tumor is found, emergency radiation treatment may be indicated.

Increased pressure within the brain may cause symptoms such as headache, lethargy, confusion, nausea, and changes in vision. Sometimes, however, the first sign of tumor spread to the brain is an epileptic seizure. Whenever increased brain pressure is detected, steroids are immediately given to reduce the pressure. When there are several areas of cancer in the brain, external radiation may be given to the entire brain. Whole brain radiation can be delivered in fractions over one to five weeks.

If only a single tumor is involved, a machine that provides tightly focused beams of radiation, such as a gamma knife, may be used to deliver the radiation. This device focuses gamma rays (a high-energy form of radiation) so that they are extremely intense at the focal point, but much less intense only a fraction of an inch away. Since a very narrow radiation beam is concentrated on a small area within the brain, a high dose of radiation can be given without fear of damaging the surrounding brain tissue.

To keep the radiation focused on the tumor, it is important that your head be kept completely still during the radiation treatment. Since it is impossible for anyone to hold perfectly still during the entire radiation treatment, a mold of your head may be made before your first radiation treatment, or a metal frame may be attached to your head to hold it in place.

Other Indications for Palliative Radiation

Radiation treatment can also be helpful when a cancer has invaded into, or is pressing on, major nerves. This is commonly seen when cancers have spread to the spine, or when gynecologic or colon cancers compress the lumbar plexus (nerves going to the legs) in the pelvis. Because dying tumor cells may swell, causing further pressure on the nerves, treatment with corticosteroids (cortisone) is often started just before beginning the radiation therapy. Cortisone treatment minimizes this swelling, helping to prevent worsening symptoms as the tumor is destroyed.

In certain instances, radiation treatment can be used to open obstructed passages in the lungs, esophagus, bile ducts, ureters (the tubes connecting the kidneys to the bladder), and blood vessels. In many cases of lung cancer, especially those occurring in the right lung, the tumor eventually obstructs a large vein, the superior vena cava. This type of obstruction prevents blood from the head, neck, and arms from returning to the heart. People with this condition, called superior vena cava syndrome, experience swelling of the upper half of the body. If allowed to progress, swelling in the neck and throat may cause difficulty breathing. Timely radiation treatment can often relieve the obstruction in a day or two.

Side Effects of Radiation Treatment

Radiation side effects occur in two phases. The first phase, which is caused by mild radiation burns to normal tissue, begins soon after the start of treatment. For example, many people experience esophageal soreness when swallowing during a course of radiation treatments to the chest. A second phase of side effects, caused by scar tissue forming in the irradiated area, may not occur for months or even years following treatment. Radiation scarring is a fairly rare complication and is usually only seen following high doses of radiation. Radiation neuropathy (nerve damage) is a very unusual late complication.

Most of the early side effects of radiation treatment are mild and easily controlled with simple therapies. The nature of the side effects is determined by the area that is irradiated. Skin reactions are usually limited to redness, irritation, itching, and sometimes superficial skin breakdown at the site that was irradiated. Radiation-induced skin reactions can be treated with topical cortisone cream, moisturizers, or topical aloe vera. Vitamin A and E ointment is also useful in promoting healing. Patients who are undergoing radiation treatment rarely, if ever, experience any skin changes that would be described as a true radiation burn.

Many people think that any exposure to radiation will cause hair loss, but this is only the case if the scalp is irradiated. When it does occur, radiation-induced hair loss is always temporary. Regrowth usually begins several weeks after completing treatment.

Radiation to the head, neck, and chest can irritate the mucous membranes lining the mouth, throat, and esophagus. The major symptoms are pain with swallowing, a constantly dry mouth, and alterations in the sense of taste. The symptoms may begin one or two weeks after starting radiation treatment and may persist for several weeks after the treatment is completed.

Mucous membrane irritation can often be treated by rinsing the mouth with weak solutions of baking soda (one or two teaspoons per quart of water). Persistent dry mouth can be treated with artificial saliva (Salivart or Xero-lube) or other lubricating agents, such as lemon-glycerin swabs. Using a medication such as pilocarpine tablets (Salagen) to increase salivary gland output can increase saliva production and prevent excessive mouth dryness.

If these treatments are not effective, your doctor can prescribe oral anesthetic solutions, such as viscous lidocaine or liquid Benadryl. Many cancer centers have their own recipes for mouth and throat rinses. One very effective remedy is a mixture of the topical anesthetic medication Diclonine with a solution of Benadryl. Some centers also add a thickening agent, such as Maalox or Carafate, to this solution so that it will coat the mucous membranes. For intractable oral pain, a 10 percent solution of cocaine mixed with a thickener (usually ground-up Carafate tablets) makes an anesthetic slurry that can be painted onto the inside of the mouth to give immediate relief.

Inflammation of the ear canals by radiation can be treated with Cortisporin eardrops. Antihistamines and decongestants can also be useful for inflammation of the middle ear or drainage from the sinuses. A few patients develop a yeast infection of the mouth and throat (thrush) after radiation. This can be treated with any of several prescription medications that kill yeast cells.

Radiation treatments involving the abdomen and pelvis may cause nausea, vomiting, diarrhea, and urinary irritation. Acute bladder irritation (radiation cystitis) is often treated with oral medications such as Pyridium. Bladder spasms may respond to antispasmodic medications such as oxybutinin or flavoxate (Ditropan, Urispas). Diarrhea usually responds to over-the-counter agents such as Pepto-Bismol or Imodium.

When the chest is exposed to high doses of radiation, the lungs may develop an inflammatory condition called radiation pneumonitis. This has many of the same symptoms as a lung infection, including a dry, hacking cough and pain during deep inspiration. Radiation pneumonitis is usually treated with corticosteroids (prednisone, 30 to 60 mg per day for three to four weeks).

Some side effects of radiation occur throughout the entire body, not just the area exposed to the treatment. These include fatigue, anorexia (loss of appetite), and nausea. These side effects are usually far less severe than those experienced with chemotherapy, and when they do occur, they are usually controlled with medications quite easily. In any case, they will stop a week or two after the radiation treatments are finished.

Palliative Chemotherapy

Palliative chemotherapy is usually not used to treat sudden increases in pain the way radiation therapy is. Rather, it is used to keep a cancer suppressed enough so that its pain remains manageable and its overall effects are limited as much as possible. When chemotherapy is used in this way to control symptoms, rather than trying to destroy all the cancer cells, the treatments can be tailored so that the side effects are much less severe.

When initially treating a cancer with chemotherapy, the oncologist often tries to maximize the intensity of the treatment; that is, use the highest tolerable doses of several chemotherapy medications given over the shortest time possible. This type of therapy maximizes tumor destruction and the possibility of cure, but also causes the most severe side effects. When using chemotherapy to treat pain, the oncologist often uses a single chemotherapy medication in a much lower dose. This type of treatment causes few (often no) unpleasant side effects. The whole point of using chemotherapy to treat pain (or any other symptom) is that the person should feel better after being treated than she did before treatment.

Using chemotherapy in this way is a fairly new development. In the past, doctors rarely gave any chemotherapy to patients unless they felt they had at least a chance to cure the cancer. The development of new types of chemotherapy with less severe side effects, along with doctors' understanding that many patients can live productive lives for years even though they have an incurable cancer, has changed this way of thinking. Doctors now prescribe chemotherapy in cases that cannot be cured, carefully tailoring the treatments to minimize the side effects it causes. The goal in such cases is to contain the cancer, slowing its growth and minimizing the pain and discomfort it causes.

This type of treatment is especially useful for patients who have relatively slow-growing cancers of the lung, prostate, breast, or colon. Many chemotherapy medications such as cyclophosphamide (Cytoxan) and etoposide (Vepesid) are available in oral forms that have relatively few side effects. An oral form of fluorouracil, the major chemotherapy for colon cancer, has recently been introduced. Vinorelbine (Navelbine), although only available in injectable form, causes few side effects when given in low doses once a week. Properly selected, these medications can often shrink these cancers, significantly reducing the cancer pain without causing significant side effects.

Breast cancer, even in advanced stages, seems particularly likely to be helped by palliative chemotherapy. Between 40 and 60 percent of women with advanced breast cancer will develop painful bone metastases during the course of the disease. For many, the bones are the only site of involvement for months or years, until the disease finally spreads to other organs. In these patients, palliative chemotherapy may relieve all the symptoms of disease for several years.

Another cancer that often responds well to palliative chemotherapy is small cell cancer of the lung. There are many reports of small cell cancers that recur after high-dose intense chemotherapy, but then go into remission on a low daily dose of an oral chemotherapy drug, such as etoposide.

Multiple myeloma, a cancer of the bone marrow that is often very painful, may also respond to intermittent doses of oral chemotherapy medications. Similarly, the pain of pancreatic cancer can sometimes be reduced by low doses of gemcitabine, while a different chemotherapy drug, mitoxantrone, can be effective in some advanced cases of prostate cancer.

When standard chemotherapy drugs are not an option or are not effective, hormonal treatments might alleviate the pain caused by certain advanced cancers. This is often the case for breast cancer, which may respond to a series of hormonal treatments even when palliative chemotherapy has failed to help. For example, many patients whose breast cancer has advanced during treatment with tamoxifen respond to treatment with hormones such as medroxyprogesterone or androgen. If hormonal therapy alone does not provide adequate relief, it may still be beneficial if combined with chemotherapy.

Research in Palliative Chemotherapy

This picture has been made even brighter by the advent of a whole new class of medications called angiostatins. These are anticancer drugs that do not directly kill cancer cells, but rather interfere with the cancer's ability to promote the growth of new blood vessels. The blood vessels that supply nutrition to tumors are not made out of the cancer cells, but rather out of normal blood vessels that were stimulated to grow by some factors secreted by the tumor.

As yet, no angiostatin has been approved for treating cancer, but studies with angiostatin medications are being conducted throughout the United States (see chapter 13 for more information about experimental trials, and Appendix F to find the locations of such trials). Angiostatins probably will not cure cancer, but will make other medications more effective. For example, if they are deprived of their nutrition supply, cancer cells are less able to repair themselves when damaged by small doses of chemotherapy or radiation. This could allow giving much smaller (and therefore less toxic) doses of chemotherapy to effectively treat cancer. Angiostatin medications may hinder cancer growth to such an extent that a person will be able to live with a slow-growing tumor for many years.

Interestingly, a medication with similar effects to angiostatin, pentosan polysulfate (Elmiron), was released in the United States nearly ten years ago for the treatment of an inflammatory disease of the bladder. There have been several reports of cancer patients obtaining some pain relief with this medication and a few reports of rapidly growing cancers that have slowed in patients taking this medication.

CHAPTER 9

Other Therapies for Pain

by Roger S. Cicala, M.D.

O ther therapies is an incredibly broad topic. Entire books are written about some of the topics that are discussed here in a few paragraphs. Obviously, there is not room to go into depth about all of them. Our major purpose here is to make sure you are aware of these treatments and know where to find more information if you are interested. We will also limit the discussion, particularly of nutritional and herbal products, to pain and symptom control. There are dozens of other books about nutrition and cancer treatment or prevention.

Finally, the information we present is based only on scientific evidence. Some pretty amazing claims are made for several of the therapies discussed here, largely based on pseudoscience. Pseudoscience is the *appearance* of scientific knowledge or facts without scientific research. The hallmark of pseudoscience is the testimonial. You've seen them on a dozen infomercials—"Mary B. of Yoohoo, Idaho, used Wonderpills and lost sixty pounds in three days." Maybe Mary did, but science would want to know what the average person lost, how many people did not lose any weight taking the pills, and how many others had a bad reaction to them. Testimonials never mention those things.

Science looks at a large number of subjects in a logical fashion. Science never uses testimonials. Rather, a scientific study would evaluate one thousand people taking Wonderpills and one thousand people taking a placebo and compare the average weight loss between the two groups. Pseudoscience marketers do not do such studies, usually because they would not want their product compared to anything.

The therapies covered in this chapter generally fall into several categories based on the scientific evidence that supports them. Some of the therapies discussed are scientifically proven to work, at least for people with certain problems or symptoms. Physical therapy, exercise, and psychotherapy all have proven benefit, for example. Some of the other therapies are not clearly proven to work, but there is some evidence that indicates they may help. Hopefully, future studies will show that these therapies actually are beneficial. Certain herbal therapies, massage therapy, and some others fall into this category. Finally, some therapies are discussed largely because they have received a lot of public attention, despite the fact that most evidence indicates they are not helpful. Magnet therapy and some of the herbal supplements fall into this category.

The Placebo Effect

Since we're going to discuss several topics for which there is no firm scientific evidence, it's important to talk about why things sometimes appear to work when they actually do not. As doctors who care for pain and other symptoms, we do not care why a treatment works in an individual. If it works, we are all for it.

We do want to know why a treatment works, though, in order to decide if it is likely to help other individuals. If a treatment only helps 10 percent of the people who use it, we might consider trying it as a last resort. However, we prefer not to waste the time and money, not to mention the risk of possible side effects, if it is not going to work 90 percent of the time. That is why doctors may seem a little cynical when they hear a testimonial, even if it's from a patient they know and trust. We have all heard hundreds of testimonials for everything from Aunt Mary's herbal tea to the latest diet fad. The vast majority of these products only work for a few individuals, however.

One thing that doctors always consider when something helps pain or other symptoms in a few individuals is the placebo effect. The placebo effect is entirely subconscious: If someone is truly convinced a treatment is going to help his symptoms, it probably will. In fact, it has been shown repeatedly that the placebo effect occurs about one-third of the time when a patient tries a new treatment. It can last for weeks or months.

If you give any treatment to a group of people, a lot of them will have the hoped-for response because of the placebo effect. A marketer can then gather testimonials from those responders and make it appear that the treatment is very effective, even if it is not. The placebo effect is one of the major reasons that doctors don't consider a treatment to be effective unless a controlled study compares the new treatment to an established treatment, with the patients "blinded" as to which treatment they receive.

Complementary and Alternative Medicines

Complementary and alternative medicines include a broad range of therapies and philosophies. These treatments are called complementary when they are used in addition to standard medical therapy. Most dietary therapies are complementary, for example. The treatments are called alternative when used instead of medical therapies. Homeopathy and chiropractic are often alternative therapies, although they can also be used as complementary therapies.

Some of the commonly used complementary or alternative therapies include psychological techniques such as relaxation or hypnosis, manual techniques like Rolfing or massage, homeopathy, vitamins or herbal products (remember, many of today's medications are simply purified herbal remedies), and acupuncture. In general, the benefits of these therapies are not as well documented as mainstream medical therapy, but there is some evidence that many of them are effective. Most of them are considered quite safe, but they sometimes cause side effects.

If you are considering an alternative or complementary therapy, you are not alone. About 10 percent of all cancer patients try at least one form of alternative therapy. Few doctors are upset about their patients using any type of complementary therapy. It is important that you let your doctor know what you are doing, however. Some alternative treatments, particularly herbal medicines and nutritional supplements, can interfere with certain medications.

Before starting the therapy, there are several questions you should ask both your regular doctor and the person providing the alternative treatment:

• What benefits can be expected from this therapy?
• What are the risks associated with this therapy?
• Do the known benefits outweigh the risks?
• What side effects can be expected?
• Will the therapy interfere with conventional treatment?
• Will the therapy be covered by health insurance?

In the majority of cases, the answer to the last question will be no. A few insurance companies do cover certain forms of alternative therapy, but most consider it experimental or unproven.

Understandably, people who suffer from cancer are often desperate. Although there are honest and honorable people who offer alternative medical treatments, there are also greedy charlatans who will take advantage of a cancer patient's desperation. Alternative treatments, for the most part, are not regulated by the Food and Drug Administration or other government agencies, which allows unscrupulous persons to make ridiculous claims for some products.

Usually, the worst that can happen to you is that you waste your time and money. However, some products can be dangerous despite the fact that they are "all natural" or "herbal." Just because a product is "natural" does not mean it is safe. Rabies virus is completely natural. So is cyanide (it is easily extracted from almond shells and peach pits). In fact, more than two hundred "completely natural" products of one type or another have been found to be extremely dangerous and were removed from the market during the last decade.

In the last few years, however, there has been an increasing oversight of alternative therapies by the government. The National Institute of Health has formed the National Center for Complementary and Alternative Medicine (NCCAM), and this agency is beginning to research and evaluate some alternative practices and therapies. They will provide what information they have about a variety of alternative medicines, herbal remedies, and complementary therapies to doctors and patients. Additionally, the Food and Drug Administration regulates some devices, such as TENS units, used for some forms of alternative therapy. Finally, the Federal Trade Commission will investigate any activities that may be fraudulent. Below is contact information for the aforementioned resources:

NCCAM Clearinghouse
P.O. Box 8218
Silver Spring, MD 20907-8218
Telephone: 1-888-644-6226 (toll-free)
TTY/TDY (for deaf and hard of hearing callers):
   1-888-644-6226 (toll-free)
http://www.nccam.nih.gov

Food and Drug Administration
5600 Fishers Lane
Rockville, MD 20857
Telephone: 1-888-463-6332 (toll-free)
http://www.fda.gov/

Federal Trade Commission
Consumer Response Center
Room 130
600 Pennsylvania Avenue, NW
Washington, DC 20580
Telephone: 1-877-382-4357 (toll-free)
TTY (for deaf and hard of hearing callers):
   (202) 326-2502
http://www.ftc.gov/

Herbal and Natural Pain Remedies

Several nutritional supplements and herbal remedies are claimed to help with pain and other uncomfortable symptoms. Most of these can be found in your local grocery store or pharmacy. You can also buy them in health food stores, although the price there is often higher. The following is not a complete list of every herbal remedy that may benefit painful conditions, just the more commonly recommended ones.

It is important to remember that herbal medicines are still medicines. They can have side effects and may have adverse interactions with other medications you may be taking. Here are some commonly used herbal medicines and their possible effects and interactions:

Echinacea may cause liver toxicity if taken in high doses or for more than eight weeks. It should not be taken with other drugs that can cause liver toxicity, such as methotrexate (chemotherapy) and keto-conazole (an antifungal medication).

Evening primrose oil may lower the seizure threshold and should be avoided by persons with seizure disorders.

Feverfew should not be taken with nonsteroidal anti-inflammatory drugs as they may interfere with each other's absorption and actions.

Feverfew, garlic, ginkgo, ginger, and *ginseng* may increase bleeding time. All should be avoided by anyone who may have low platelet counts after chemotherapy.

Ginseng may cause headache, tremors, and anxiety in patients treated with phenelzine sulfate. It should not be used by persons taking estrogens or corticosteroids because of possible additive effects. It should not be taken by diabetics because it can increase blood sugar and may interfere with digoxin blood levels.

Hawthorn may interfere with digoxin blood levels.

Kava should not be taken at the same time as tranquilizers because of increased sedation.

Kelp may interfere with thyroid replacement therapies.

Licorice can offset the pharmacological effect of some diuretics and interfere with digoxin blood levels.

St. John's wort probably should not be taken by persons taking selective serotonin reuptake inhibitors (SSRIs).

Uzara root may interfere with digoxin blood levels.

Valerian should not be used with tranquilizers or alcohol because excessive sedation may occur.

Mental and Emotional Remedies

Ginkgo

Ginkgo, or *Ginkgo biloba,* refers to an extract from the leaves of the ginkgo tree, the oldest surviving species of tree on earth. For years, herbalists have claimed that ginkgo can treat many conditions associated with aging, including memory loss. Ginkgo is also claimed to help the fatigue and difficulty concentrating that some cancer patients experience. It may also have antidepressant effects.

Medical studies have shown that the active ingredient in ginkgo, platelet activation factor (PAF), helps restore blood flow through the brains of people with cerebral vascular disease. Several European studies have shown improved memory, thinking, and reasoning ability as measured by standardized tests in persons taking ginkgo. More recently, a yearlong study published in the *Journal of the American Medical Association* also found that patients receiving ginkgo had improved mental function.

It should be noted that even in the most optimistic study, the effect of ginkgo was small. It is important to remember that herbal medicines like ginkgo are still medicines—they have side effects. Ginkgo can interfere with blood clotting and may cause allergic reactions, and some people report headaches or nausea when taking it.

Melatonin

Melatonin is a natural hormone secreted by the pineal gland in the brain. Its major known effect is in regulating the circadian or sleep-wake cycle, and it is widely used as an over-the-counter treatment for insomnia. The sleep-wake cycle of the body not only affects sleep, but also regulates several other functions including the daily changes in body temperature and blood levels of some hormones.

There is some scientific evidence that taking melatonin at bedtime helps restore a more normal sleep-wake cycle in patients who do not sleep well at night, but are drowsy during the day. Most studies report that about one-third to one-half of such people improve after taking melatonin. A few people find it actually makes their sleep patterns worse, however.

Melatonin is sold over-the-counter in the United States, but it is regulated as a medication and requires a prescription in Europe. Almost nothing is known about interactions between melatonin and other drugs and diseases, but because melatonin is a potent natural hormone, it may cause problems, particularly in persons who have hormone-secreting tumors. Although a trial of melatonin is probably worthwhile for persons with severely disturbed sleep, it should be stopped at the first sign of worsening symptoms.

St. John's Wort (Hypericum)

St. John's wort has been recommended for the treatment of depression, and several scientific studies suggest it is effective. St. John's wort has an excellent safety record and appears to cause few side effects or adverse reactions. Photosensitivity (sensitivity to sunlight) occurs in a few people taking St. John's wort. In those cases, the photosensitivity is usually mild. However, people undergoing radiation therapy should probably avoid St. John's wort until their treatment is complete. St. John's wort may interfere with the absorption of iron, so it should not be taken by people who need iron supplements.

Valerian (Valerianae officinalis)

Valerian is an herb that some people claim relieves restlessness and aids sleep. It also is said to reduce anxiety and nervous conditions, improve concentration, and perhaps reduce pain. Valerian is available in capsules, pills, juice, teas, liquid concentrate, and as the fresh herb. The active ingredients, called valepotriates, are removed to some extent in processing, so some people claim the fresh herb is more effective than the other forms.

Because valepotriates can have toxic effects in high concentrations, valerian should not be taken to excess. It can also increase the effect of sedative medications and the sedative effect of opioids (pain medications). For this reason, it is a good idea to begin taking valerian at a low dose and increase the dose gradually. The usual dose is two to three grams of herb or extract (about two tablespoons of juice) taken once or twice a day.

A few people experience odd feelings of being separated from their surroundings when taking valerian. More common side effects include headache, nausea, and intestinal cramps. Occasionally, the herb has an effect opposite to the one expected, causing restlessness, excitability, and insomnia, similar to drinking too much coffee.

Remedies for Joint Problems and Bone Pain

Cartilage and Chondroitin Sulfate

Shark cartilage products are widely used in the United States for the prevention and treatment of cancer. They are also used for other painful conditions including arthritis, psoriasis, and muscular pain. About fifty thousand Americans use cartilage supplements regularly, and more than forty brand names of shark cartilage products are sold in the United States. The major components of shark cartilage are proteins and calcium salts. Chondroitin sulfate, one of the proteins found in cartilage, is sometimes sold separately.

Cartilage compounds are marketed as dietary supplements, so they do not require Food and Drug Administration evaluation or approval. Also, there are no specific quality control requirements for cartilage or other dietary supplements. This lack of regulation means there is no guarantee that any claims made about these products are accurate. There are not even any guarantees that the package contents actually are cartilage, or that the product is pure and safe to use.

Several European studies have demonstrated that chondroitin sulfate, an ingredient found in cartilage, improves joint mobility and reduces pain in arthritis sufferers. There is some evidence that either cartilage or chondroitin may also help patients who have significant joint pain from other causes, including the joint pain that sometimes develops after radiation or chemotherapy. However, chondroitin must be taken for at least several weeks to show any beneficial effect.

Most of the attention given to cartilage, however, involves its use as a cancer-treating supplement, not as a pain supplement. Since the 1970s, the use of shark cartilage as a cancer treatment and preventive has been heavily marketed because of the belief that cartilaginous fish (sharks, skates, and rays) do not get cancer. However, this is not true; several studies by marine biologists have found that many cartilaginous fish captured over the years do have cancers such as melanomas and soft-tissue sarcomas. Several large clinical studies looked for any effect that shark cartilage might have on treating or preventing cancer. So far, every study has concluded that shark cartilage has no beneficial effect for preventing or treating cancer.

Glucosamine Sulfate

Glucosamine sulfate is the major component in chondroitin. That is, chondroitin sulfate is made up of many repeating units of glucosamine sulfate linked together. By chemically breaking these links, free glucosamine sulfate is obtained. The major advantage to doing so is that glucosamine is a much smaller molecule than chondroitin and therefore is better absorbed into the body. Only about 15 percent of an oral dose of chondroitin is absorbed into the body (the rest just passes through the intestines), whereas more than 90 percent of oral glucosamine is absorbed.

Advocates also claim that the glucosamine molecule will pass into the joints better than the chondroitin molecule. Not surprisingly, the health food companies that make glucosamine claim that it is far superior to chondroitin for relieving joint pain. Like chondroitin, however, it must be taken for several weeks to show any benefit. In the standard dose of 500 mg taken three times daily, glucosamine appears to be quite safe. It may interfere with the absorption of other medications taken at the same time, however, so it should not be taken within an hour of other medications.

White Willow Bark

White willow bark has been used by Native North Americans as a pain reliever for more than a thousand years. There is strong evidence that it is helpful for the pain of headaches, backaches, and arthritis, and that it helps lower fevers. The reason it is effective is quite simple. One of the major ingredients of white willow bark is salicin, which is the precursor to the active ingredient in aspirin. Like aspirin, however, willow bark may cause stomach problems if taken regularly.

Arnica

Arnica is derived from several species of the daisylike flower arnica, which grows in the high mountains of western North America. Pure arnica is toxic when ingested and should never be taken internally. Health food stores sell very dilute oral doses of arnica, as well as arnica ointments, and claim that it is effective for muscle pains, stiffness, swelling, and local tenderness. One scientific study, done in Great Britain in 1991, did find that arnica relieved stiffness in patients with muscle pain.

Arnica ointment has been reported to cause skin irritation in some persons. It can also be toxic if applied over broken skin.

Antioxidants

Antioxidants are chemicals that neutralize free radicals—molecules with unpaired electrons that can damage various tissues within the body. The body constantly produces free radicals during normal metabolism. The amount of free radicals increases after exposure to radiation, burns, cigarette smoke, certain drugs, alcohol, and during infection. Because antioxidants can neutralize the free radicals, they may have several beneficial effects, including reducing the pain caused by inflammation.

Since the pain associated with cancer often involves inflammation, antioxidants may help reduce cancer pain. The effect is probably slight, but all antioxidants are extremely safe if taken in reasonable doses. The antioxidants currently available are vitamins C and E, beta-carotene, selenium, bioflavonoids, bioflavanols, and manganese. There are many brands of antioxidant pills available that combine most of these antioxidants in a single capsule.

Vitamin E

Vitamin E prevents free radical damage and has several beneficial effects. Some good scientific studies indicate it may also help reduce muscle soreness after exercise. Other studies, although less scientific, hint that it may help reduce muscle soreness from many different causes, presumably by reducing muscle inflammation. For this reason, it is sometimes recommended for those people who have significant muscle pain after chemotherapy or radiation treatments.

Pycnogenol

Pycnogenol, at the time of this writing, is a "hot topic" on the herbal medicine circuit and in health food stores. It is a bioflavonoid derived from the bark of certain French pine trees and from grape seeds. A lot of scientific evidence has found that pycnogenol is very good at neutralizing free radicals. In fact, it is twenty to forty times more potent as an antioxidant than either vitamin E or vitamin C.

Pycnogenol marketers claim the substance works for almost everything, including pain, arthritis, heart disease, emphysema, high blood pressure, cancer, and anything else you care to name. Because it is claimed to stimulate the immune system, it is often taken as a supplement by cancer patients. There is fairly good scientific evidence that it does help reduce the pain associated with inflammation, which is a significant part of the pain associated with certain types of cancer.

The usual dose is 100 to 200 mg taken three times a day. Because pycnogenol stays in the body for some time, some people recommend taking 200-mg doses for the first week to "saturate" the body, and then reducing the dose to 100 mg. Adverse side effects are rare, but nausea and stomach irritation is sometimes reported. A few people have developed an allergic skin rash after taking it for several days.

Nausea and Vomiting Supplements

Ginger

Ginger has been recommended for many years as a treatment for intestinal spasms and cramps. There is also some good evidence that it reduces nausea and vomiting. Scientifically, it has been studied and found effective for nausea associated with pregnancy, motion sickness, and certain diseases. It has not been specifically studied for nausea associated with chemotherapy, but anecdotal reports state that it is sometimes helpful. Ginger root powder is available in capsules. The usual dose is one 250-mg capsule four times a day. Fresh ginger root can also be made into tea, which some claim to be more effective. There are some claims that ginger is also effective as an anti-inflammatory supplement, but no studies support this, however.

Green Tea
Green tea has been advocated as a treatment for nausea and intestinal cramps in patients undergoing chemotherapy. It clearly seems to settle the stomach of some patients during chemotherapy. It has also been advocated as an antioxidant. Green tea is the least processed and freshest of teas, and it does have significant antioxidant activity, which more processed teas do not have. Some of the antioxidant activity comes from the large amounts of vitamin C it contains, but it also contains other antioxidant chemicals. Unfortunately, some health food advocates recommend about ten cups of green tea a day for antioxidant activity. Since green tea contains about half the amount of caffeine that coffee does, this will result in a significant caffeine dose. Caffeine can worsen insomnia, pain, and anxiety, so green tea may not be a good choice as an antioxidant for cancer patients.

Psychotherapies

Many, if not most, cancer patients can benefit from short-term psychotherapy or by learning some psychologic techniques. It is not surprising that a number of different types of psychotherapy have clearly been shown to reduce stress, anxiety, and depression in patients undergoing cancer treatment. You may be surprised to learn that many studies have shown such therapies can also help the immune system work better, reduce nausea after chemotherapy, and reduce pain. There are even some studies that show psychotherapies can improve life expectancy, at least in certain types of cancer.

The types of psychotherapy we are referring to do not involve lying on a couch and telling someone about your childhood. Rather, they involve a number of different techniques provided by psychiatrists, psychologists, nurses, social workers, and lay therapists. In its simplest form, psychotherapy provides emotional support and information while helping patients learn some coping skills that will help them adapt to the crisis of having cancer. Many cancer centers offer such programs to every single patient. More in-depth or individual psychotherapy is available for patients with severe pain, clinical depression, or other problems. Family members, who are almost as likely to suffer emotional difficulties as the patient, can also benefit from psychotherapy.

Although we cannot teach the techniques involved in this chapter, we do want to make sure you know some of the therapies that are available. Some are very simple, but in almost every case, having someone work with you for an hour or two will be much more effective than trying to do it on your own. If you are interested, your oncologist can make a referral for you to obtain treatment.

Pastoral counseling or support from your own minister can provide many of the benefits achieved by psychotherapies, particularly since many ministers are trained in some of these techniques. Ministers or hospital chaplains can also be a wonderful source of information on community resources, as well as providing spiritual care and support for patients and their families.

Distraction and Reframing

Distraction simply involves focusing on things other than unpleasant symptoms, such as pain, nausea, or sadness. Everyone uses some internal and external distractions. Internal distractions can be praying or thinking "I can handle this, I've done it before." External distractions include listening to music, watching television, reading, or talking to friends.

Distraction techniques that therapists can suggest include thinking exercises and mental puzzles, rhythmic massage, or using a visual focal point. Some self-hypnosis techniques are quite easy to learn and can often relieve mild pain or manage brief episodes of severe pain, such as occur with some procedures. Several daily meditation and inspirational books just for cancer patients are available that provide excellent tools for distraction.

A related technique, reframing, teaches patients to monitor and evaluate negative thoughts and images and replace them with ones that are more positive. For example, patients who are preoccupied with a fear of pain can rehearse positive statements or write lists of positives to read over when such thoughts occur.

Humor Therapy

Humor therapy is not really a psychotherapy at all (most psychologists I know are not very funny), but actually a form of distraction therapy. It has been shown in several studies, however, that watching comedy videos, telling jokes, or even playing practical jokes cannot only dramatically improve a patient's mood, but relieves pain and reduces nausea following chemotherapy. Some centers make it a point to play comedy tapes during chemotherapy sessions. Others recommend watching some form of comedy at least twice a week.

Meditation and Relaxation Techniques

Many people already know some meditation techniques. If not, there are several simple techniques that can be learned in two or three group sessions. Meditation is especially useful to help calm and relax oneself before and after chemotherapy or other treatments. It can also be a great way to get "back on track" if feelings of hopelessness or anxiety become overwhelming at certain points during the day. Most patients who use meditation say that it works best for them when they reserve time for two or three brief meditation sessions at intervals during their day.

Relaxation therapy is similar to meditation, but some people prefer relaxation techniques, especially those who are having difficulty concentrating because of stress or anxiety. The most commonly used form of relaxation therapy is an audiotaped session that a person can play at any time. Some people use them at regular intervals during the day, while others use them on an as-needed basis. There are some excellent mass-produced relaxation tapes. Most cancer centers keep some available for their patients to borrow. The best tapes, however, are made for a person's individual use by a psychologist or other trained therapist. These tapes can include specific relaxation methods that are most effective for that particular person.

A related technique called guided imagery helps people to relax and become calm by thinking of real or imagined places where they feel completely at ease. Guided imagery may also use soft music, readings, or other aids to help people reach a comfortable frame of mind. The technique can be practiced silently or may be aided by a recorded tape. As with relaxation therapy, guided imagery tapes made particularly for the patient are often more effective than mass-produced tapes. Many centers offer guided imagery groups to teach the technique to cancer patients.

Family and Patient Support

There are dozens of different kinds of support groups. Groups can involve patients, family members, or both. They may focus on specific types of cancer, specific symptoms (depression, nausea, pain), different stages of cancer (in remission, just diagnosed), and have specific agendas (education, emotional support). Some groups are directed by a professional; others are simply gatherings of people with similar problems or interests. Most support groups meet in a physical location every week or so, but there are groups that meet via Internet chat rooms or E-mail. Additionally, several national and regional services provide individual support by linking cancer patients to a cancer survivor of similar background.

We strongly encourage every cancer patient to try some type of support group for at least a little while. Dozens of studies have clearly demonstrated that both patients and family members who are involved with support groups have less depression, milder symptoms, far less anxiety, and (for patients) slightly longer life expectancies than those who aren't. Each person must decide what type of support group or groups would be most beneficial for them. To help you find what is available, Appendixes D and E provide telephone numbers and Internet addresses for many different support groups.

Physical Therapies

Physical therapy is generally used to help restore physical strength and functioning after injury or surgery. Physical therapists can also provide a lot of pain relief for patients with musculoskeletal (involving the bones and muscles) pain, some types of neuropathic pain, and sympathetically mediated pain. Physical therapists have experience with different pain-relieving techniques and often advise doctors about treatments that may benefit a patient they are working with. Many of the techniques they use, such as ultrasound stimulation, require special equipment and a person trained in using it. Other techniques, such as exercise, range of motion therapy, and mechanical stimulation, can be done just as effectively by the patient himself, perhaps with help from a family member.

Exercise

Exercise is important for both treating and preventing pain in cancer patients. Routine exercise strengthens weak muscles, mobilizes stiff joints, helps restore coordination and balance, improves circulation, and reduces swelling. Even very simple things, like frequently changing position and moving all the joints through a full range of motion, can be helpful. In one study, pain was reduced in 86 percent of bedridden patients by simply changing their positions every hour or so. Even 25 percent of otherwise active cancer patients reported reduced pain after beginning an exercise program.

It does not require a hospital setting and special therapists to start exercising. Many local YMCAs and other community organizations have organized exercise programs for recovering cancer patients. For people who have difficulty walking, structured exercise programs performed in a swimming pool can provide dramatic relief of joint and muscle aches and pains. Pool therapy can even be performed by persons who are at risk of pathologic fracture because of metastatic tumors that have invaded their bones.

When patients are too severely ill to exercise, family members should learn how to perform range of motion exercises and massage. Often, a physical therapist can make a few home visits to demonstrate these techniques. When performed regularly, simply moving all the joints through the normal range of motion can reduce swelling and pain in a bedridden patient. It will also preserve muscle length and joint motion during periods of severe illness, making recovery much easier. However, range of motion exercises should not be carried out in a limb with a fracture, or if movement increases pain severely. All forms of exercise that involve weight bearing should be avoided if there is a likelihood of pathologic fracture or tumor invasion.

Positioning and Movement

Proper positioning is another simple technique that can relieve pain in bedridden patients. Many bedridden patients cannot position themselves comfortably without help. Proper position involves keeping the body correctly aligned with no twists in the back or limbs. Joints should not be kept completely extended, but rather slightly flexed, which will minimize swelling of the extremity. If any area of the body has paralysis or severe weakness, a padded splint can prevent contractures (permanent shortening of tendons and muscles) and spasms. Skin condition should also be monitored, and the patient should be helped to roll or turn frequently so that pressure sores do not develop.

Immobilization or restriction of movement is often used to manage episodes of acute pain, to stabilize fractures, or to prevent fractures in patients with bone metastasis. Physical therapists can make home visits to provide supportive devices such as adjustable elastic braces and splints to maintain optimal body alignment.

However, prolonged immobilization should be avoided whenever possible by performing range of motion therapy several times a day. For example, a patient may need to have her shoulder immobilized because of a pathologic fracture. Range of motion can still be performed on her elbow, wrist, and fingers so that these joints do not become stiff.

Massage and Vibration

Massage helps relax and increase circulation to the areas massaged. This can reduce the pain from muscle aches, lessen swelling, and relieve joint pain associated with immobility. Depending on the area involved and the tenderness of the skin, soft stroking, firm kneading, or rubbing with rhythmic, circular motions may give the best results. An alcohol-free lotion can reduce friction, minimizing skin tenderness during the massage. Warming the lotion for a few seconds in a microwave may make its application more comfortable. Massage should not be considered an alternative to exercise or range of motion, however.

Mechanical massagers or infrared heating massagers can help increase superficial circulation and may make it easier for the person giving the massage. Vibrators often relieve the pain of damaged nerves or peripheral neuropathy (nerve damage of the feet and hands) that sometimes results from chemotherapy. *One word of caution:* Infrared heating devices should not be used in areas that have recently received radiation, as they may cause burns.

Ice and Heat

Applying heat or cold to painful areas can sometimes reduce pain dramatically. Heat increases blood flow to the skin, decreases blood flow to the underlying muscles, and reduces joint stiffness. Heat can be applied by hot packs, hot water bottles, electric heating pads (dry or moist), commercially available chemical and gel packs, and immersion in a tub or basin. Devices that deliver deep heat, such as diathermy, infrared, and ultrasound devices, can also be used, but should not be placed directly over a cancer site.

Heat should be applied for at least thirty minutes, but can remain in place longer. When used for more than thirty minutes, however, the skin should be inspected several times to make sure there is no burning. Hot packs should always be wrapped in a towel or cloth to prevent burns. If the patient has any nerve damage or numbness in the area, more layers of protection should be used, since skin burning is more likely. Heat should never be used in areas that have recently undergone radiation therapy because these areas are very likely to burn.

Cold causes vasoconstriction, reduces inflammation and swelling in injured tissues, and reduces some types of pain, particularly burning pain. Although most people do not realize it, cold probably relieves muscle spasms better than heat does. Ice packs and frozen chemical gel packs are the simplest ways to apply cold. Cold packs should be sealed to prevent dripping and wrapped in cloth so that they are not uncomfortable. The pack should be soft enough to conform to body tissues in the area. Cold should generally not be applied for as long a time as heat; fifteen minutes is usually sufficient.

Although cooling will increase joint range of motion and relieve muscle spasm in most conditions, in a few cases it increases joint stiffness and muscle spasm. If that occurs, cold therapy should not be used. Cold should not be applied to any area that has been damaged by radiation therapy. It also should not be used in areas with vascular problems, such as in a limb with peripheral vascular disease. Patients who have certain connective tissue diseases such as lupus may actually have more pain if they use cold.

Acupuncture

Acupuncture has been practiced in China for more than five thousand years. It has been used to treat many conditions, but for cancer patients, the relief of pain, nausea, and vomiting are the most important. Acupuncturists place very thin stainless steel or copper needles just under the skin, and then stimulate the needles by gently twisting, heating, or applying a weak electrical current to them. This usually produces a tingling sensation, or one similar to a mosquito bite. Acupressure (applying pressure to designated points instead of inserting needles) may have similar effects.

According to a panel of experts at a National Institutes of Health Consensus Conference in November 1997, acupuncture is considered "somewhat effective" in the management of nausea and vomiting associated with chemotherapy. The conference also concluded it might have some effect in controlling postoperative pain. Much of the evidence in support of acupuncture is anecdotal (based on individual patients' reports of benefit) rather than from controlled studies. However, scientific studies have shown that acupuncture causes the release of natural opioids that can reduce the perception of pain. Anatomic studies have shown that the acupoints (locations where acupuncturists insert needles) have a greater concentration of nerve endings than do other locations on the body.

If you decide to try acupuncture, only visit an acupuncturist who is licensed (all fifty states license acupuncturists). Also, never have an acupuncture session if your blood count is low, as may happen after chemotherapy. This could place you at very high risk of infection or bleeding.

Biofeedback

Biofeedback can teach a person how to control many of the involuntary functions of the body. Among other things, people can learn to control heart rate, blood pressure, muscle tension, and even emotions. Biofeedback uses monitoring electrodes that are placed on the body or scalp and connected to amplifiers and a computer. The computer uses lights, sound, or both to show the intensity of whatever function the patient wishes to control. During biofeedback sessions, a therapist helps the patient learn how to mentally control and change the signals, thereby controlling and changing the function in question.

Biofeedback is most commonly used to teach people how to relax spasmed muscles and reduce the muscle tension associated with stress. This undoubtedly reduces pain and improves the quality of life for those who are successful. Biofeedback has the advantages of being noninvasive, inexpensive, and safe. It usually requires between five and fifteen sessions before a person achieves effective control.

TENS

TENS stands for transcutaneous (meaning across the skin) electrical nerve stimulation. A TENS device applies a controlled, low-voltage electrical current through electrodes placed on the skin. Theoretically, the current may interfere with the ability of nerves to transmit pain signals to the spinal cord and the brain. A different theory claims TENS stimulation "overrides" the pain signal in the spinal cord. Even after several decades of research, however, it still is not clear if TENS provides any better pain relief than a placebo. The device is easy to try and simple to use, however, and some people have had excellent relief of mild to moderate pain using TENS.

CHAPTER 10

Nerve Blocks and Nerve Destruction

*by David Leggett, M.D., and
Claudio Andrés Feler, M.D., F.A.C.S.*

To a physician practicing pain management, the term *nerve block* is not very specific. There are actually many different types of nerve blocks, each used for slightly different reasons. In the broadest sense, a nerve block simply means injecting a medication near a nerve that reduces or stops the ability of the nerve to transmit information to the brain.

Nerve blocks were first used for local or regional anesthesia before the turn of the twentieth century. These medications blocked nerve tissue from conducting messages back and forth, so that surgical procedures could be performed without requiring general anesthesia. The shot that numbs your gums at the dentist's office is technically a nerve block. This type of nerve block has only a temporary effect, usually lasting a few hours at most.

Many years ago, anesthesiologists and other doctors began trying to treat various chronically painful conditions with nerve blocks. Obviously, the few hours of relief that were obtained with local anesthetics were not very beneficial to patients who hurt constantly, so the doctors began using other medications in addition to, or in place of, the local anesthetic. The term *nerve block* continued to be used, however, even if no anesthetic was injected and the nerve signals never became blocked.

Today, a variety of very different procedures are all referred to as nerve blocks. Many different medications can be injected including narcotics, steroids, antihypertension medications, anti-inflammatory medications, and others. Some of these medications are also used as intraspinal medications and are discussed more fully in chapter 11.

In addition to varying the medication injected, nerve blocks also vary according to exactly where in the body the medication is placed. The location of the injection is generally divided into three categories: central, peripheral, and sympathetic. Central blocks involve injections near the spine. Depending on the exact location of the injection, central blocks can also affect other structures such as bones, ligaments, intervertebral discs (the pad between each bone in the back), the joints of the back, and the spinal cord and spinal nerves. Peripheral nerve blocks involve injections near various nerves outside the spinal column. This could include nerves traveling to the legs, arms, face, or head. Sympathetic blocks involve injections of the sympathetic (unconscious) nerves. (See chapter 1 for a discussion of pain arising from the sympathetic nerves.)

Nerve Blocks for Spinal Pain

Cancer frequently causes back and spine pain both directly and indirectly. The most common direct cause of spine pain is the spread of the tumor to the vertebrae (bones of the spine). Although any type of cancer can spread to the spine, certain types, such as breast, colon, and prostate cancers, are more likely to metastasize to the vertebrae. In a few instances, the sudden onset of back pain is the first indication that a patient has cancer.

Metastatic cancer causes pain by deforming the bone and stretching or irritating nerves in a tissue layer called the periosteum, which covers the bone. The cancer may also weaken a vertebra to the point that it collapses on itself, resulting in a compression fracture. In some cases, the cancer can invade or compress the spinal cord or its nerve roots, resulting in pain that mimics that of a ruptured disc.

Certain types of cancer can cause back pain without actually invading the spine. For example, abdominal tumors such as pancreatic cancer can invade tissues behind the abdomen. The distension and inflammation of the muscles and nerves compressed by the tumor result in pain in the lower and middle back regions. Cancers of the kidney can cause similar effects.

The indirect effects of cancer probably cause as many cases of back pain in cancer patients as those caused by spread of the cancer to the spine. Cancer patients often experience considerable fatigue both from the cancer and from treatments like radiation and chemotherapy. Patients are often forced to curtail physical activity and may become bedridden. This diminished physical activity increases the likelihood that muscle and connective tissue in and around the spinal column will become irritated and inflamed, resulting in substantial back or neck pain.

Spinal injections are a mainstay in the management of both back and neck pain caused by the direct and indirect effects of cancer. They can benefit patients suffering from spine pain caused by metastatic invasion of the spine, and those whose pain results from indirect effects such as muscle weakness.

Epidural Blocks

The most common nerve block performed for the treatment of back or neck pain is undoubtedly the injection of cortisone into the epidural space of the spine, commonly called an epidural block. The epidural space is located within the bones of the spine, but outside the tough tissue covering the spinal cord, which is called the dura. "Epi" is the Latin root for outside, hence in an epidural block the medication is injected outside the dura. A spinal tap or spinal block is an injection into the spinal fluid that lies under the dura and is therefore referred to as a subdural injection.

Local anesthetic medication injected epidurally can provide anesthesia for surgery or labor pains and can control postoperative pain. The epidural injection of dilute local anesthetic solution containing cortisone (also called corticosteroids) can reduce nerve inflammation to improve chronic back or neck pain.

In the management of cancer-related pain, epidural injections can take two forms: a single injection or continuous infusion. The single or one-time injection is most common. A needle is placed in the proper location, and a quantity of medication is injected followed by removal of the needle. The entire procedure takes only a few minutes.

The continuous infusion epidural is used only in certain specific conditions. A needle is inserted exactly as it would be for a one-time injection. After needle placement, however, a very small catheter (medically, catheter means a soft tube) is threaded through the needle into the epidural space. The needle is then withdrawn, but the catheter is left in the epidural space for anywhere from several days to several weeks, depending on the circumstances and method of insertion.

From a technical standpoint, epidural injections are relatively safe and painless. An intravenous infusion is started in all patients, both for safety and to administer sedation when needed. The amount of sedation varies according to the individual patient and the physician performing the procedure, but the goal is to provide patient comfort without creating complete unresponsiveness. This procedure is usually performed with the patient lying face down (prone), but in some cases the patient may remain sitting for the procedure.

In most pain treatment practices, the use of fluoroscopy (real-time X ray) to confirm proper placement of the needle is routine; however, its use is not mandatory. The fluoroscope is used to show the relevant bony anatomy of the spine, and the insertion point is marked on the skin. The skin is then prepped with an iodine solution, and the insertion site is anesthetized with local anesthetic via a very small needle. The epidural needle is then inserted and directed to the proper location and depth using the X ray for guidance. Once proper placement is achieved, the medication is injected (or the catheter inserted), the needle is removed, and the procedure is complete. The average epidural injection takes ten to twenty minutes to accomplish. Most patients can return home within an hour of completing the procedure.

Not all patients can undergo spinal injections, and some people require extra precautions before attempting the procedure. The two most common contraindications for spinal injection are infection and poor clotting of the blood. Infections anywhere in the body increase the possibility of the epidural needle becoming contaminated with bacteria, thus spreading the infection to the epidural space. Infection in the epidural space can cause meningitis or an epidural abscess. Since the epidural space is close to the spinal nerves and spinal cord, any infection in this area could have devastating consequences if not treated immediately. While the occurrence of an epidural abscess is very rare, the presence of an infection increases the risk enough so that the procedure should be delayed until the infection is fully treated.

Anticoagulation, the reduced ability of the blood to clot, can in rare cases lead to bleeding in the epidural space and the development of an epidural hematoma (pool of blood in the tissue). The epidural space contains many small veins, and the needle sometimes punctures one of the veins during the procedure. In patients whose blood clots normally, the puncture heals naturally like any small wound. If the blood does not clot normally, the vein may continue to leak blood into the epidural space until a hematoma has formed. The hematoma can exert pressure on the nerves and spinal cord, possibly causing permanent damage or requiring a major surgical procedure to relieve the pressure.

The other possible complications of epidural injection are all temporary. These include headache and backache. These complications are infrequent and almost always resolve within a day or two. A mild weakness or numbness is expected to occur from the local anesthetic, but will only last an hour or two. Overall, the risk of epidural injections is extremely low, and for most patients the potential benefits far outweigh the risks.

Other Blocks Near the Spine

There are several other injections used in the management of spine pain. These include spinal facet injections (injections into the joints between vertebrae), selective nerve root injections (injection into a single nerve as it leaves the spine), and intradiscal injections (injections into the intervertebral discs). Each of these techniques can be helpful for treating certain specific causes of back pain, but none of them is particularly useful for treating cancer pain.

Intrathecal (also called subdural) injections are used to place medication into the spinal fluid. Placing a needle into the subdural space to obtain a sample of spinal fluid for analysis is fairly common for patients with certain types of cancer, but injecting medication into this space is done infrequently. Constant infusions of opioids (narcotics) into the spinal fluid is sometimes used for pain control, however (see chapter 12).

Patients whose pain originates from pancreatic cancer may benefit from a special type of injection performed near the spine called a celiac (pronounced "see-lee-ack") plexus block. The celiac plexus is a collection of nerves that lies in front of the spine, near the aorta. This plexus transmits much of the pain information from the upper gastrointestinal system and the organs of the abdomen, including the pancreas.

Many patients with pancreatic cancer experience pain as their tumors invade the soft tissue structures near the pancreas. Blocking or deadening the celiac plexus may substantially reduce the pain. Patients who obtain good but short-lived pain relief from a local anesthetic injection are often candidates for a longer lasting neurolytic (nerve destroying) injection (discussed later in this chapter).

A celiac plexus block can be performed by any of several techniques, but from the patient's standpoint the procedure is similar to that experienced during an epidural block. Most physicians perform the block using two needles, one advanced from each side of the back, instead of the single needle used for an epidural block. The needles also are placed deeper into the body than is needed for an epidural block. For this reason, patients usually are sedated rather heavily for a celiac plexus block. They are also likely to have muscle soreness in their backs for several days after the procedure.

Patients who experience pain from pelvic or perineal (the floor of the pelvis) tumors may benefit from a superior hypogastric plexus block (to show you how silly medical terminology is, this literally translates as "upper lower stomach plexus"). This procedure is similar to a celiac plexus block, although it is performed in the lowest part of the back near the sacrum (tailbone). This injection may also be done using a neurolytic technique to provide long-lasting pain control, but this is not performed very often.

The complication rates for both the celiac plexus and superior hypogastric plexus blocks are somewhat higher than that of an epidural block. However, when performed with fluoroscopy (X-ray guidance), significant complications are very rare. Since the pain of pancreatic and pelvic cancers can be difficult to control with medication alone, the relief provided by these blocks can be particularly important.

Blocks for Peripheral Nerve Pain

Peripheral nerves are the major nerves that connect the spinal cord to various body regions. Because the nerves follow well-mapped paths throughout the body, it is possible to inject local anesthetics near the nerve at various locations, making a portion of the body insensitive. Many people have experienced peripheral nerve injections when a dentist numbs a tooth, or a physician sews up a small cut using local anesthesia.

Peripheral nerve injections are not used for the management of abdominal and lower extremity cancer pain very frequently, because epidural and subdural injections work so well for pain originating in these areas. However, peripheral nerve injections can be vitally important for managing cancer pain in the head and neck region. They are also used occasionally for pain originating from the chest wall and arms.

Cancers of the face, head, and neck can be extremely painful, since these areas have a very dense supply of nerves and are very sensitive to painful stimulation. Because the nerves of the head and face do not travel through the spinal cord (instead, these nerves pass directly though the skull to the brainstem), epidural and spinal blocks are of no benefit for pain above the neck. When pain medication cannot control the pain of head and neck cancer, injection of an anesthetic (sometimes with cortisone) near the nerves that are transmitting the pain can be very helpful.

A variety of different nerve blocks can be used in the head and neck region. The various indications for each block are somewhat technical, but generally they are classified as diagnostic, prognostic, or therapeutic. Diagnostic blocks use short-acting anesthetics (lidocaine is commonly used) to determine exactly which nerves are carrying the pain signals to the brain. In some cases, it is obvious which nerves are involved by the location of the pain, so a diagnostic block may not be needed.

Once the exact nerves involved have been determined, a prognostic block is performed to let the patient experience the potential consequences of a permanent neurolytic (nerve-destroying) injection. This block uses a longer acting local anesthetic that provides six to twenty-four hours of relief. It may seem silly to perform a prognostic block (many patients want to skip it and simply have the nerve destroyed permanently), but it is vitally important. Peripheral nerve blocks do not simply stop pain; they also result in areas of numbness and weakness within the distribution of that nerve (remember the effect some of those dental injections have on your lips). For some patients, a constant sensation of numbness can be more disabling than the pain that the injection is treating. Additionally, nerve blocks near the face may paralyze facial muscles, causing difficulties with chewing, swallowing, and speech. A prognostic block lets the patient determine how satisfied he might be with a permanent nerve block.

Therapeutic injections, sometimes called neurolytic (pronounced "new-row-lit-ick") blocks, involve injecting substances such as alcohol or phenol that chemically injure the nerve. A single neurolytic block can result in several months of pain relief. These nerve destruction procedures are discussed more thoroughly later in this chapter.

Although head and neck pain is the most common indication for peripheral nerve blocks, these procedures are sometimes used in other body regions. For example, patients with metastasis to a rib often experience severe pain in the chest wall. Injection of local anesthetic or a longer acting agent near the intercostal nerve (the nerve running just beneath each rib) can provide pain relief in the affected area without causing any problems other than numbness in that area. Relief of chest wall pain is particularly important, since it allows better breathing. It can even help patients sleep by eliminating the pain that results when they roll over in bed.

Peripheral nerve blocks may also be used when a tumor compresses a peripheral nerve. This sometimes occurs with tumors of the upper lung, which can press the brachial plexus (the network of nerves passing over the chest on their way to the arm and hand). In some cases, an injection of cortisone near the nerve may reduce the swelling around the tumor enough to relieve the nerve compression.

Blocks for Sympathetically Mediated Pain

As discussed in chapter 1, some cancer patients develop severe pain transmitted through the sympathetic nervous system (part of the nervous system controlling unconscious functions of the body, such as sweating or regulating blood flow through the tissues). The cause of sympathetic pain is not clearly understood, but it causes devastating pain if not treated effectively. Patients with bony metastases in the extremities and those who have received radiation therapy are somewhat more likely to develop sympathetically mediated pain, but it has been caused by many other conditions.

There is no test that clearly determines if a patient's pain is originating from the sympathetic nervous system. Some symptoms, such as a burning character to the pain, hypersensitivity of the skin in the affected area, and red or bluish discoloration, may hint that the pain is originating from the sympathetic nervous system. The condition may be the cause of pain that does not respond well to opioid (narcotic) medications.

When sympathetically mediated pain is suspected, a block of the sympathetic nerves can help to confirm the diagnosis and to treat the condition. Many different nerve blocks can be used for the treatment of sympathetically mediated pain. The most common are lumbar sympathetic blocks, stellate ganglion blocks, and Bier blocks.

Lumbar Sympathetic Blocks

A lumbar sympathetic block is used to diagnose and treat sympathetic pain originating from the foot or leg. From the patient's point of view, a lumbar sympathetic block is similar to an epidural block, with the needle placed in the lower back while the patient lies on her stomach, but the block is administered quite differently. When performing a lumbar sympathetic block, the doctor injects the anesthetic outside the vertebral column, which is the location of the sympathetic nerves.

When it is performed properly, a lumbar sympathetic block stops all activity in the sympathetic nerves to one leg, but does not interfere with the voluntary nerves. Since the voluntary nerves still function normally, there is no loss of sensation or weakness after the block. Because the sympathetic nerves do not function, the leg often becomes pink and warm as the blood vessels in the area dilate. If the block provides pain relief, that gives strong evidence that the sympathetic nervous system is involved in the pain. If the pain remains the same, then the sympathetic nervous system is probably not involved.

The pain relief following a lumbar sympathetic block is temporary; it may last for up to twelve to forty-eight hours. A series of three or four lumbar sympathetic blocks performed once every two or three days may give long-lasting relief. If the original block is not beneficial, however, there is no reason to repeat it.

When performed under fluoroscopic (X-ray) guidance, lumbar sympathetic blocks are considered very safe. Major complications are exceedingly rare, although some soreness in the muscles of the back should be expected for a day or two following the procedure.

Stellate Ganglion Blocks

For sympathetically mediated pain of the arm, head, or neck, a stellate ganglion block is performed. The stellate ganglion, also called the cervicothoracic ganglion, is a collection of nerve connections located outside the spine near the base of the neck. The sympathetic nerves to the head, arm, and upper chest all originate from this area.

As with a lumbar sympathetic block, the injection of local anesthetic in this area stops activity in the sympathetic nerves without affecting motor or sensory nerves. Substantial pain improvement after a stellate ganglion block is evidence that the pain is mediated by the sympathetic nervous system. If the pain is relieved, a series of blocks is performed as described above.

Stellate ganglion injections require placing a needle into the base of the neck from the front. The patient is usually lying on his back during the injection, but a few doctors prefer to perform the procedure with the patient sitting up. Because the doctor can identify the stellate ganglion by touch, using X ray is uncommon unless the patient is substantially overweight or has had extensive neck surgery in the past. The procedure can be performed quite quickly (often in only a minute or two) and typically gives very little discomfort.

Stellate ganglion injections are relatively safe in the hands of experienced physicians, but even in the best hands, some complications are possible. The stellate ganglion is located very close to important structures in the neck, including the spinal nerve roots and the vertebral artery (an artery that passes up the neck to the base of the skull, eventually providing blood to the brainstem). It is possible for some of the local anesthetic injected during the procedure to reach either of these structures. Accidental injection into the vertebral artery could cause a seizure and loss of consciousness. Injection near a nerve root could cause the anesthetic to block the higher parts of the spinal cord and brain, which also causes unconsciousness.

Bier Blocks

Bier blocks are a different method sometimes used to relieve sympathetically mediated pain. Bier blocks are simpler to perform and perhaps less uncomfortable than stellate and lumbar sympathetic blocks. They do have some limitations, however. For example, Bier blocks can only be used in the lower portion of the arm or leg (below the elbow or knee, respectively). Additionally, they cannot be used to diagnose sympathetically mediated pain, because the block also affects the voluntary nerves.

The procedure itself is quite simple. An intravenous catheter is placed into the hand or foot of the painful limb. The arm or leg is then tightly wrapped in an elastic bandage, starting at the hand or foot and working toward the body, effectively squeezing most of the blood out of the limb. A blood pressure cuff or tourniquet is inflated to prevent the blood from returning to the extremity, and the rubber bandage is removed. After the tourniquet has been inflated, a large quantity of local anesthetic (and possibly other medication) is injected through the IV catheter. The medication travels throughout the veins and is absorbed by the tissues in the extremity, including the branches of the sympathetic nerves.

Within a few minutes, the entire arm or leg becomes numb and remains so until the tourniquet is released (usually twenty to thirty minutes).

Many studies using various combinations of local anesthetics and anti-inflammatory, antiseizure, and cardiac medications have been attempted with this technique. Although results are mixed, and no one medication is clearly most effective, some patients do get substantial improvement in sympathetically mediated pain after treatment with Bier blocks.

Nerve Destruction Procedures

A nerve destructive procedure is essentially any technique that damages a nerve so that it can no longer function. There are several different methods used to damage a nerve, including thermal (heat or cold), electrical, chemical, and surgical. To treat cancer pain, the goal is to damage a nerve so that it can no longer transmit pain messages to the spinal cord. Theoretically, this would relieve all the pain coming from the area served by that nerve.

On the surface, it would appear that nerve destruction procedures would be an ideal way to relieve cancer pain coming from a single area. Unfortunately, like so many issues in modern medicine, it is not that simple. It is natural to assume that nerve destruction is the equivalent of a permanent nerve block, but this is not so. The actual duration of a nerve destruction procedure may only last a few weeks and usually lasts less than six months. This impermanence occurs for two simple reasons: nerve repair and cancer progression.

Visualize a single nerve cell as a yo-yo dangling from a finger. The actual yo-yo is the nerve cell body and the string is the nerve fiber. In a human the cell body is located in or near the spinal cord, and the nerve fiber extends out into the arm, leg, chest, or face. When a doctor destroys a nerve in your arm or leg, he is actually damaging a large number of nerve fibers. The cell body remains undamaged in the spinal cord.

After the nerve fiber is damaged, the cell bodies attempt to repair the injury by growing a new nerve fiber along the path of the nerve. The growth process is both very slow and very chaotic. Because a single peripheral nerve contains thousands of fibers, the individual nerve fiber usually does not reconnect to its original location exactly. In some cases, a nerve fiber may reconnect to a slightly different area. In other cases, the new nerve fibers are unable to travel down the nerve and instead form a tangled ball-like formation within scar tissue, called a neuroma (pronounced "new-rome-ah"). As abnormal connections or neuromas are formed, the patient may begin to experience pain again. This may or may not be similar to the original pain, and over time, it may even become more severe than the original pain.

In addition to nerve regrowth, there is the issue of cancer progression. If it is not cured, cancer eventually spreads, invading new structures. If the tumor grows into areas not covered by the original nerve destruction procedure, the pain obviously will return.

Despite these limitations, nerve destruction procedures can be very useful in certain situations. Deciding when such procedures should be used involves considering the life expectancy of the patient and the possibility of cancer cure, understanding the nerve pathways carrying the pain signal, and the patient's ability to tolerate the predicted side effects. Nerve destruction should only be considered when the pain cannot be well controlled by using oral medications or other pain-relieving therapies. If there is a significant chance that the painful tumor can be cured, or at least reduced with radiation or chemotherapy, these methods should be tried before considering nerve destruction.

Nerve destruction is often very appropriate for patients who are in the terminal stages of cancer. Patients with advanced cancer often suffer severe pain that may require such high doses of pain medication that they are always sedated. A nerve destruction procedure may allow the medication dose to be dramatically reduced, letting the affected person remain comfortable, yet alert enough to enjoy time with his loved ones. Since nerve destruction procedures often last for several months, a single procedure may provide good pain relief for the life expectancy of a person with advanced cancer. Of course, predicting the duration of pain relief and life expectancy is at best educated guesswork, so repeat nerve destruction procedures may be necessary.

Since nerve destruction procedures only provide relief to a certain area of the body, they are not useful for patients suffering widespread pain involving large portions of their bodies. However, even such persons may have one or two areas that are much worse than pain in other areas. Targeting these areas with nerve destruction techniques may reduce the pain level sufficiently to allow oral medications to provide effective relief for the remaining pain.

In any case in which a nerve destruction procedure is being considered, a prognostic nerve block with local anesthetic should be performed first, so the patient can decide if a nerve destruction procedure is worthwhile. Some people find the numbness or weakness to be worse than the pain itself. Weakness, in particular, is often unacceptable to individuals who are already struggling to maintain some degree of personal freedom and self-care.

Nerve Destruction for Abdominal and Pelvic Cancer

Despite its drawbacks, nerve destruction can be a very valuable tool for controlling pain in properly selected patients. Most patients will undergo a trial injection with local anesthetics prior to the actual nerve destruction procedure. If they do not receive pain relief with the local anesthetic block, there is no reason to believe that the neurolytic injection will give long-term benefit.

Certain cancers located within the abdomen or pelvis, such as pancreatic cancer, cancer of the cervix, or bladder cancer, respond very well to nerve destruction, because the nerves carrying pain signals from these locations are fairly easy to destroy. For example, most of the pain caused by pancreatic cancer is routed through a single nerve structure called the celiac plexus that is located between the spine and the abdomen.

The celiac plexus is a network of sensory nerves from the internal organs; it carries little or no motor information. When the plexus is blocked, patients with pancreatic cancer usually experience excellent pain relief without any numbness or weakness. Nerve destruction is performed almost identically to the standard celiac plexus block described earlier. Instead of injecting local anesthetic, however, a neurolytic (nerve-damaging) chemical is used. Pure alcohol or phenol is the most commonly used chemical.

After destruction of the celiac plexus, most patients usually have at least 50 percent of their pain relieved. There may be some transient side effects, such as reduced blood pressure or diarrhea, but these usually subside after twenty-four to seventy-two hours. The beneficial effects of the procedure usually last about three months, but may last as long as six months. If the pain returns or intensifies, the procedure may be repeated, but repeated neurolytic injections are often less effective than the first block. This is because scar tissue forms around the plexus after the first injection. The scar tissue prevents the neurolytic chemical from spreading into the tissues with repeat injections.

Certain lower abdominal and pelvic cancers, such as bladder or uterine cancer, may also be treated with neurolytic injection. The procedure used, although very similar to a celiac plexus injection, targets a different group of nerves called the hypogastric plexus. This plexus is located in front of the lowest bones of the spine. The success rate of hypogastric plexus block is somewhat less than celiac plexus block, but the complication rate of the procedure is low.

Peripheral Nerve Destruction

Unfortunately, most peripheral nerves carry both motor and sensory information. A permanent block with alcohol or phenol will destroy at least some of the motor nerve fibers, causing weakness or even complete paralysis. For patients with advanced cancer, this loss of motor function may be unimportant when compared to achieving better pain control. However, some individuals may find the persistent numbness or weakness unacceptable. For this reason, it is crucial that patients receive a trial of local anesthetic injections prior to undergoing a more permanent procedure.

The most common locations for peripheral neurolytic injections are the face, neck, and rib cage. Facial injections may provide the most dramatic pain relief, but can also have the most significant side effects because of motor weakness. Depending on the exact nerves involved, side effects could include difficulty speaking, chewing, and swallowing. In a few rare cases, severe skin damage or complete loss of jaw muscle control has occurred.

Injection of the chest wall is also very helpful and is associated with far fewer side effects. There is a small (less than 1 percent) chance that a chest wall injection could cause a collapsed lung (pneumothorax). If a collapsed lung occurs, it might be necessary to insert a small tube through the chest wall to reexpand the lung, and a hospital stay of several days could be required. This is certainly not a minor complication, but almost all patients who suffer lung collapse recover without any significant permanent injury. As with most nerve destruction procedures, the risk is slight when compared to the potential pain relief that could be obtained.

Some peripheral nerves, particularly the ones in the chest wall, can be blocked with a special technique called cyroanalgesia, which means freezing the nerve. Cryoanalgesia is performed just like other nerve blocks, but instead of injecting medication, a special needle-shaped probe that can rapidly freeze tissues is used. Cryoanalgesia destroys the nerve, although not as completely as a neurolytic injection. It can provide weeks or even months of pain relief and can be repeated more easily than chemical injection, since it causes less scarring. Cryoanalgesia equipment is bulky and costly, however, so it is not always available. Because the probes are somewhat larger than regular needles, it is not appropriate for some of the other nerve destruction procedures.

Neurosurgical Destruction of Spinal Cord Nerve Tracts

Historically, ablative (destructive; pronounced "ah-blate-iv") neurosurgical procedures were often performed on the spinal cord to relieve the most severe types of cancer pain. These interventions are used much less frequently today, having been replaced by better medications, nerve blocks, and intraspinal medications (see chapter 11). Nevertheless, a few patients are still appropriate candidates for these ablative operations.

Many different ablative procedures can be used to treat cancer pain. Perhaps the most frequently used historically, and still the most useful today, is the cordotomy. In this operation, a small part of the spinal cord is cut surgically or burned with a radio frequency (similar to microwave) needle. The part of the spinal cord that is destroyed is called the lateral spinothalamic tract. The lateral spinothalamic tract (see chapter 1) is the bundle of nerve fibers that carries painful sensations up the spinal cord to the part of the brain called the thalamus. The procedure can be performed through a very small incision, so general anesthesia is not usually required.

Cordotomy is most effective for pain originating in the leg and hip on one side of the body. It is less effective at relieving pain originating in the arm or the trunk. Cordotomy is also much more effective for controlling somatic pain and usually not effective against neuropathic pain (see chapter 1). After the procedure has been done, the patient will have some numbness on the side of the body on which the procedure was performed.

The location of the spinothalamic tract within the spinal cord must be estimated when a cordotomy is performed. Although this estimation can be done quite accurately (to a small fraction of an inch), the spinal cord is densely packed with other fiber tracts involved in other functions. It is possible that some of these other tracts could be injured during cordotomy, resulting in difficulty controlling bladder or bowel function, or weakness of the leg on the involved side. These complications are more common when cordotomy is performed on both sides of the spinal cord, as must be done if the pain involves both sides of the body.

Because of the potential complications, cordotomy is usually performed only for patients who either have leg pain on only one side, or who already have lost control of their bowels and bladder. Finally, a significant number of patients will experience return of their pain after six or eight months. For this reason, the procedure is usually reserved for terminal patients.

Summary

Cautions Regarding Nerve Blocks

The use of nerve blocks remains an important tool for treating cancer pain, especially for terminal patients. In the hands of qualified physicians, the injections are safe and potentially very effective. Unfortunately, even the most skilled physician cannot avoid every complication. It is critical that patients and their families take an active role in deciding if a procedure is right for them.

Before undergoing a nerve block procedure, be sure to discuss it fully with your doctor. Take the time to understand the possible risks and weigh those against the possible benefits. Do not consent to a procedure unless you are comfortable, or at least fully informed, as to what might happen. However, do not expect guarantees! No physician can or should promise a certain outcome.

Do not be afraid to ask for your physician's qualifications and certifications. Is he board certified? Does he have special training and experience in performing the procedure? It is always appropriate to ask doctors how many times they have experienced a particular complication, and how they handle it when it occurs. Such questions do not antagonize a good doctor, who will want you to be fully aware of any risks. If you are uncomfortable with the answers you receive, do not hesitate to ask for a second opinion.

In most cases, you will be instructed about various do's and don'ts for before and after your injection. *Do not ignore these instructions.* The most common reason for canceling a procedure is the patient's failure to follow the eating guidelines. *If you are told not to eat for eight hours before your block then please do not eat!* Complications from nerve blocks are rare, and in most cases easy to treat, but the worst complications occur in patients who have had food or liquids before the procedure.

One of the most common complications of a nerve block or the sedation that may be given is a brief loss of consciousness. This usually has no consequences, but if a person with food or liquid in her stomach becomes unconscious, the stomach contents could go down the windpipe and into the lungs. This can cause a very dangerous and possible lethal lung injury.

Most doctors do want you to take your medicines with a small sip of water, however. If you are not sure, call and ask. Following your doctor's preblock and postblock instructions will minimize your risk and improve the chances for a good result.

Expectations and Failures

Nerve blocks, just like pain medication, chemotherapy, and radiation, give doctors a very powerful tool to treat cancer pain. Just like those other therapies, however, they do not work for every single patient. There are a number of possible reasons why a nerve block may not help. Sometimes the patient expected total relief following the injection, and this is rarely possible. In other cases, the block simply "missed" and did not make the nerve numb. If your doctor suspects this has happened, she may recommend repeating the procedure.

In other cases, there were causes of pain that the block could not relieve. This may occur when the tumor involves areas supplied by more than one nerve, or if the individual's anatomy is a bit different from normal, meaning a different nerve than expected carries the pain signal. In such cases, it may be possible to do a different nerve block in an attempt to relieve the pain. In other cases, a nerve block simply may not be possible.

PART III

Advanced Treatments for Cancer Pain

CHAPTER 11

Intraspinal Treatments for Cancer Pain

by Claudio Andrés Feler, M.D., F.A.C.S.

D
elivering medications and implanting electronic devices into the spine (not into the spinal cord, but inside the bones of the spine, near the spinal cord) have become some of the most powerful tools we have to treat cancer pain. They are just that, however, powerful tools. The techniques discussed in this chapter are not miracle cures, and they are not appropriate for every cancer patient.

This is one part of the book that you probably should not read until you have gone through the chapters in Part I that discuss the various types of pain. The reason for this is simple: The techniques we are going to discuss are each appropriate only for pain originating from certain causes. If you have not read about the difference between neuropathic pain and visceral pain, for example, you probably will not follow the discussion in this chapter very easily.

With that mentioned, it is very important to realize that one person's pain is not physically the same as another's. The pain may not be transmitted to the brain by the same pathways, and the pain signal probably does not use the same neurotransmitters. Almost every person who has cancer pain will suffer from somatic pain (see chapter 1), the "normal" pain caused by tissue injury, or things that might cause tissue injury. Oral pain medications, such as morphine, relieve this type of pain most effectively.

Many cancer patients, especially those who undergo extensive treatments for their cancers and those whose cancer progresses, also suffer from other types of pain. Over time, a slowly progressing cancer invades various tissues, damaging body organs and structures. Treatments such as radiation, chemotherapy, or surgery may themselves have caused harm to nervous system tissues, causing neuropathic pain (see chapter 1). These types of pain usually do not respond to morphine or the other opioid pain medications.

Cancer patients who have neuropathic pain almost always have somatic or visceral pain, too. The treatment of pain in these cases is more complicated and difficult, because there is generally no single treatment that will relieve both types of pain. In many cases, several different combinations of medication will be tried in an attempt to control the pain. If a successful medical combination cannot be found, or if the side effects of the medications are too severe, the procedures discussed in this chapter might be appropriate.

Not every cancer patient is a potential candidate for these procedures. Below is a list of general requirements that must be present to consider neurosurgical interventions for cancer pain control. This list is not absolute; there are certainly some exceptions that might still be treated with the procedures we are about to discuss. The list does provide some general guidelines, however.

1. After multiple trials of oral medications:
   a. All effective oral medications cause intolerable side effects, or
   b. Pain is poorly relieved by oral medications, or
   c. Medication costs would be reduced significantly by the procedure.
2. The patient has adequate function of the immune system to fight infection.
3. The costs associated with the device are covered by insurance or affordable to the patient.
4. A trial of the technique has relieved pain (for those techniques involving permanent implantation).

Traditionally, neurosurgeons have used procedures that destroy parts of the nervous system to help relieve cancer pain. These procedures remain useful for some patients (see chapter 10), but all are associated with a significant number of complications and risks. More recently, nondestructive techniques have been developed, largely in hopes that the newer procedures could avoid the complications of those destructive procedures. As a general rule, physicians work under the ancient principle of *primum non nocere* (Latin for "first, do no harm"). Thus, nondestructive operations are almost always recommended first. In a few circumstances, however, they may not be the best choice.

The different techniques of using nondestructive procedures to alter pain are all grouped under the name *neuromodulation*. The two most common types of neuromodulation are intraspinal drug delivery (infusing drugs near the spinal cord) and neurostimulation (implanting electronic stimulators near the spinal cord or a peripheral nerve). Intraspinal drug infusions allow medications to be absorbed directly into the spinal cord.

When administered this way, the medications can work much more effectively than when they are spread throughout the entire body. This method may also avoid many of the side effects that the medications can cause. Neurostimulation uses computer-generated electrical signals to interfere with the ability of the nerves and the spinal cord to transmit pain messages to the brain.

Generally, these methods do not completely relieve all of a patient's pain. They reduce the pain to levels that can be easily managed by medications or that are bearable to the patient. Each technique is most appropriate in certain situations, and unlikely to help in others.

Intraspinal Drug Administration

Two techniques have been used to deliver medications near the spinal cord: epidural catheters and implanted infusion pumps. They are not used interchangeably; they have quite different indications and uses, as shown in Table 11.1. Of the two, implanted pumps are far more useful for long-term care, while epidural catheters are generally used for, at most, weeks or a few months.

TABLE 11.1

Differences Between Epidural Catheters and Implanted Pumps

	Epidural Catheter	Implanted Pump
Dose used	High	Low
External catheter	Yes	No
Medication absorbed into body	High	Low/none
Patient/family injects medicine	Usually	No
Life expectancy	Less than 3 months	More than 3 months

In either case, intraspinal drug administration can provide excellent pain relief from somatic pain, particularly the pain of bone invasion by metastatic cancer. It is also quite effective for treating visceral pain, such as that arising from tumors of the kidney, pancreas, or liver. It is generally not as effective against neuropathic pain, but some new medication combinations may make it helpful for that condition. Finally, because of the location of the catheter within the spinal column, intraspinal drug systems work best for pain involving the legs or trunk. In some circumstances, it can work well for pain originating from the head and neck, but it loses many of its advantages when used in this location.

Some patients who get good relief from oral opioid medications but are unable to tolerate the side effects of opioids are also excellent candidates for intraspinal pumps. Giving medications intraspinally can dramatically reduce constipation, sedation, and confusion. It may or may not reduce the severity of nausea and vomiting, however.

Epidural Catheters

The epidural catheters (catheter simply means a soft tube) used for cancer pain treatment differ very little from the catheters inserted for pain relief during childbirth or after surgery. The tip of the catheter is placed inside the bones of the spine, but outside the sack of fluid that contains the spinal cord. To insert the catheter, a hollow needle is inserted through the skin and placed in the proper location using X-ray guidance. The catheter is then passed through the needle and the needle is withdrawn, leaving the catheter in place.

Medications given through the epidural catheter are absorbed into the nerve roots as they pass out of the spine and, to a lesser degree, absorbed into the spinal fluid and spinal cord. Fairly high doses of pain medication must be given through epidural catheters, although the dose is far less than that needed by mouth. The dose is high enough, however, that some of the medicine will be absorbed into the bloodstream and distributed throughout the body.

Opioid medication given through epidural catheters can often provide much better pain relief than medication taken by mouth or injected into a muscle or vein. Local anesthetic medications can also be given through the catheter and may provide much better pain relief than opioid medications. The medications can be continuously infused into the catheter using a pump similar to the one used to give intravenous fluids.

The major advantages of an epidural catheter are that it is simple, inexpensive, and easy to insert without surgery. There are several disadvantages, however. Usually, the catheter is brought out through the skin and connected to an injection port or an infusion pump. This is not uncomfortable (the catheter is not any larger than that used for an IV), but it can be inconvenient for some people. Because the catheter exits through a small hole in the skin, there is a low but constant risk that infection may develop. Finally, because larger doses of medication are required (compared to an implanted pump), the monthly cost of medication is usually higher than that of an implanted intraspinal pump.

Epidural catheters are usually used to treat patients during the last stages of cancer. In this situation, the low cost of the device and the ability to insert it without surgery is much more important than the higher cost of medications. The risk of infection is limited in such situations because the time of use is shorter, and the inconvenience of being connected to an infusion pump is usually less important.

Drug Infusion Pumps

Implanted drug infusion pumps (also called morphine pumps or intraspinal pumps) have been available since the 1980s. Unlike an epidural catheter, a drug pump is implanted completely under the skin. It contains a reservoir for medication that is filled at the doctor's office every few weeks (ranging from three to eight weeks, depending on the medication and dosage used). The pump infuses medication twenty-four hours a day. (See Figure 11.1) Some pumps allow the infusion rate to vary, so that a higher dose can be given at night, for example. Most pumps can be adjusted at the doctor's office to increase the rate of infusion as conditions change.

The greatest benefit of the implanted pump is its ability to provide pain relief without many of the common side effects of opioids, such as sedation, confusion, and constipation. This is due to the fact that when medicines are infused directly over the spinal cord, very small quantities of drug provide the same or better pain relief than very large amounts of the same medicine given by mouth or intravenously. For example, a routine oral dose of morphine for a patient with severe pain may be 300 mg per day. The same patient may get better relief with only 5 mg of morphine per day infused into the spinal fluid. Because the drug absorbs directly into the spinal cord, the brain is not usually affected by the medicine, meaning there is little sedation.

Intraspinal infusion devices have their own set of problems, or at least potential problems. The most common problems (which are still quite rare) involve simple medication reactions and allergies, not any trouble with the pumps themselves. However, the pumps are mechanical devices, and although it is very rare, they can malfunction. Mechanical or electrical malfunction of the device could cause an overdose, or obstruction of the catheter could prevent the medication from entering the spinal fluid. Of course, as with any implanted device, there is the possibility of infection developing. Infection is much less likely with an implanted pump than with an epidural catheter, however.

The most commonly used infusion pumps run on an internal battery that usually lasts for several years. If the battery becomes depleted (or if the device stops working for any other reason), no medication enters the

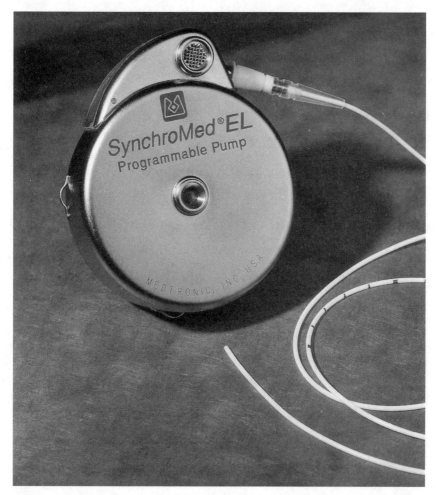

Figure 11.1: An implantable intraspinal infusion pump (Medtronics SynchroMed EL) attached to the catheter that is used to infuse medications into the spine. (Photo is courtesy of Medtronic, Inc.)

spinal fluid and the patient could go into physical withdrawal. The other type of infusion pump uses a freon-charged pressure infusion system. These devices do not need a battery. The infusion rate changes with major changes in the ambient air pressure (this just means that you can't go climb a mountain or scuba dive) and temperature. In spite of the real risk in their use, infusion pumps have been used for many years by thousands of patients. They have proven to be very safe devices.

Pump Trials

It's important to remember that the pump itself is not the therapy. The therapy is the infused medication that provides the pain relief. No matter how appropriate intraspinal infusion therapy seems for an individual patient, we can never be certain that the medications will work without side effects. We also will not know which medication or combination of medications will work best until they have actually been tried. Although morphine sulfate is the only drug currently FDA approved for treatment of pain by intraspinal infusion, many other drugs are effective when infused this way (FDA approval is not necessary to use an existing drug in a different way). Other medications that have been used for intraspinal infusion include Dilaudid, fentanyl, sufentanil, Demerol, clonidine, baclofen, Marcaine, and ketamine.

Each patient is unique and has a slightly different response to any given medication. Any of these medications may provide relief to a particular patient, or a combination of several may be necessary before good pain relief is obtained. Some patients will have no side effects from any of the medications; other patients may react to almost all of them. A few individuals will not get any relief from any of the intraspinal medications.

Because of the different drug options available, and to be certain that intraspinal drug infusion is likely to work well, a trial of the therapy must be done before the device is permanently implanted. This involves administering test doses of the drug or drugs that are thought most likely to relieve the person's pain.

Usually, a trial of one medication or one combination of medications is done each day. The patient spends the day doing normal activities and decides how beneficial each medication is. These test doses can be given by repeated spinal injections, or a catheter can be implanted in the spine so that the patient does not have to go through daily spinal injections. It is extremely important for the patient to give an accurate evaluation of each medication trial. These test doses not only determine if the pump should be implanted, but also which medications are most likely to work well.

Once it has been decided that the therapy will be effective, the infusion pump is surgically placed in the patient. This procedure can be done simply using intravenous sedation and local anesthesia; a general anesthetic is not required. Although many patients want to be "put to sleep" for the procedure, local anesthesia is usually considered much safer for a patient with chronic illness such as cancer. The pump is usually filled with medication during surgery, and the infusion started immediately afterward. Assuming there are no complications (there usually are not), patients usually stay in the hospital for one to two days after undergoing pump implantation.

After discharge from the hospital, it is often necessary to adjust the infusion rate of the pump or the type of medication used. In a few cases, this may be needed every week for the first month or so, but usually it is required less frequently. If the pump is battery powered, such as the Medtronics SynchroMed, adjustment of the amount of drug infused is done by simply changing the device's computer program (no needle sticks required). If the pump is the freon-powered variety, such as the Arrow M-3000, the drug itself will have to be removed and replaced with a different concentration anytime an adjustment is needed (yes, a needle stick). Once a few adjustments have fine-tuned the medication, further adjustments are needed only every few months, or even less frequently.

Regardless of which type of pump has been implanted, the pump will eventually run out of medicine and need to be refilled. In either case, the pump is refilled by injecting the medication through the skin into the reservoir of the pump. At that time, the pump may also be adjusted, if needed. If a battery-powered pump has been selected, the battery will deplete about every five years, on the average. Then the entire pump must be replaced in a minor surgical procedure. In spite of the fact that a battery will eventually wear out, the management of a patient with a multiprogrammable pump is much easier and more pleasant for the patient. For this reason, we rarely recommend freon-based pumps.

Neurostimulation

Neurostimulation for the treatment of painful conditions dates back to the 1960s when neurosurgeons used modified cardiac pacemakers to treat painful conditions affecting the lower back. Initial attempts at placing these sorts of devices were first carried out at the level of nerve roots, later near the spinal cord, and ultimately in the brain. Initial results were poor, in part due to the poor quality of the devices then available and also due to the limited understanding of physical causes of various painful conditions. Over the past thirty years, these devices have changed significantly. The devices themselves are now much more powerful, and the electrodes and electronic systems more complex and flexible. Similarly, there have been significant advances in the quality and power of the battery systems used to power these devices. These changes have made it possible to use neurostimulation effectively for the treatment of cancer pain.

In sharp contrast to drug infusion devices (intraspinal pumps), stimulators benefit patients with neuropathic pain (see chapter 1) the most. This type of pain often feels like a constant burning or aching sensation, sometimes associated with sudden shooting or electrical shock pains. Often the patient's skin becomes very sensitive to light touch or cold. Sometimes the patient feels as if the area is numb, yet painful at the same time. Patients with neuropathic pain usually do not get good relief with medications but can often benefit from neurostimulation.

Just as a test is done when considering an implanted infusion device, a neurostimulator must be tested before it is permanently implanted. Performing a trial requires a minor surgical procedure, not much different from having an epidural nerve block done. (See chapter 10.) It can be done in several different ways, but the essence of the test is to place a small wire electrode (Figure 11.2) over the spinal cord, either through a needle or via a small surgical incision made under local anesthesia. This lead is attached to an external electronic generator and a trial of stimulation is begun in the operating room.

During the trial, the best location for placing the leads is determined by turning on the stimulator and moving the electrode to a position in the patient's spine that causes a tingling sensation in the same area as the pain. Once the electrode has been placed, a temporary electrical wire that connects the electrode to the external generator is brought out through the skin. The generator contains a tiny computer that creates the electrical signals. The doctor or an assistant programs the computer to generate electrical signals that feel comfortable to the patient (often a mild tingling or massagelike sensation) and that relieve the pain. The

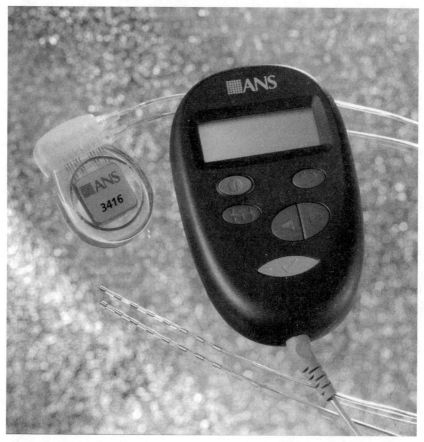

Figure 11.2. An implantable neurostimulator attached to paired spinal electrodes. (Courtesy of and permission granted by Advanced Neuromodulation Systems, Inc.)

trial continues for a period of days, allowing the patient to decide whether or not neurostimulation helps control her pain.

If the trial provides good pain relief, the patient returns to the operating room to have a permanent generator placed under the skin. (If the therapy was unsuccessful, the electrode may have to be removed in the operating room or may simply be pulled out through the skin, depending on the type of electrode used.) After the generator is implanted, the patient typically stays in the hospital for one more night. The device can be used immediately, but as the surgical incisions heal, it may move slightly, requiring it to be reprogrammed. Rarely, the electrodes may move enough that it requires several adjustments to obtain a final program that works well.

Complications from spinal cord stimulation are rare, but infections, spinal fluid leaks, and even spinal cord injuries have been reported. Except for the possible movement of an electrode, which usually requires simply reprogramming the device, all these complications are unusual. The advantages of neurostimulation far outweigh the risks in appropriate patients. Since no medication is involved, there is no possibility of medication allergy or side effects. Most importantly, for certain types of pain there is no other therapy as effective as neurostimulation.

Certain types of tumors may grow quite quickly, resulting in pain that rapidly spreads to other parts of the body. To effectively treat patients with these kinds of tumors, it is necessary to plan ahead and presume that the pain will spread. This means implanting a device that can later be reprogrammed to cover the increased area of pain. Not all spinal cord stimulating devices can allow for such a degree of reprogramming, so it is important to discuss device selection with the doctor performing the procedure before a permanent implantation is done. It is this phenomenon that most limits the use of spinal cord stimulation in patients with cancer pain. Nonetheless, for an appropriate candidate, there is no safer therapy available.

Summary

Although medical management can control most cancer pain for most patients most of the time, patients with certain types of pain cannot obtain adequate relief with any combination of medications. These patients should consider intraspinal interventions for pain treatment. The specific treatment choice depends on several factors, so it must be individualized to the patient. Important factors include the cause of the patient's pain, its location, the underlying source of the pain, the likelihood of significant spread of the pain location, and the life expectancy of the patient. When these decisions are made properly, the condition of a patient and his comfort can usually be greatly improved by the use of these devices.

CHAPTER 12

Pain Treatment for Specific Situations

by Roger S. Cicala, M.D.

Much of what is discussed in this chapter is also discussed elsewhere in the book, but by necessity is scattered about. That may make it difficult to find what exactly can be done about your specific kind of pain. And so, this chapter summarizes or reviews cancer pain treatment in general, but also focuses specifically on the treatment of the more common pain syndromes cancer patients suffer. For each condition, we will try to summarize which of the various kinds of treatment are most helpful, and refer you back to other parts of the book that may discuss those treatments more thoroughly.

We will make a couple of assumptions. The first is that you have read enough of the book to understand the source of your pain, or that your doctor has already explained the exact causes of your pain. If you know, for example, that you have neuropathic pain in your ribs from radiation therapy and aching pain in your legs from a tumor involving the bone, this chapter should tell you what specific treatments are most likely to help. On the other hand, if you just know you hurt really bad but are not sure why, then you should definitely read Part I before jumping in here.

The other assumption we will make in this chapter is that you have already tried the routine treatments for cancer pain. Just to make certain that routine treatments have been attempted, we will start with a section that discusses the World Health Organization's protocol for the general treatment of cancer pain. When we begin discussing the different painful syndromes (a group of symptoms with a common cause), however, we will not repeat that you should first try anti-inflammatory and long-acting opioid medications. We will assume that has already been attempted and that further treatment is needed.

Finally, note that many times cancer patients fall into the "if-then" trap. One of the most common is "If my pain were relieved, then I wouldn't _____ ." You can fill in the blank with many different things: feel depressed, stay awake all night, yell at my spouse, be so tired, and so forth. In other words, if the pain were gone, the other problems would all be gone, too.

That is often the case, but not always. In some cases, the depression or anxiety can actually be worsening the pain. As discussed in chapter 1, pain and suffering are often two different things. Remember that there are usually things you can do about the other symptoms that are separate from treating the pain problem. You might go back and read chapters 4 and 9 to see if you might be missing some helpful therapies.

Protocols for the General Treatment of Cancer Pain

In 1986, the World Health Organization (WHO) published guidelines for cancer pain management based on the "three-step ladder." Every cancer patient, regardless of the exact cause and source of his pain, should be started on at least the first two steps of this ladder before considering other therapies.

The essential concepts in the WHO approach include taking the medications by mouth, by the clock, and by the ladder. This means taking the drugs as scheduled (not when you really hurt; they do not work as well that way) and in a logical progression. That is, we do not destroy nerves or implant morphine pumps until we have done the best we can with the routine, oral pain medications.

You might be surprised (or maybe you wouldn't) at how many patients want to undergo major, risky, pain-relieving procedures when the first medication (or two) is not working well. The stepwise, logical approach usually works much better in the long run, however.

The first step in the WHO ladder is the use of nonsteroidal anti-inflammatory drugs (NSAIDs) and other nonopioid medications for pain control. These medications may be all that is required for some cancer patients with mild pain. It usually takes only a few days to tell if an anti-inflammatory medication is going to provide enough pain relief.

The second step is the addition of an opioid medication when the first step is not adequate to control pain. This step is a bit more complex and takes longer to try. Different opioids must be tried to find which ones work best for an individual. Then opioids of stronger potency and longer duration are tried until adequate pain control is achieved, or side effects have become unacceptable. It often takes several weeks or more to decide if oral opioids will adequately control the pain.

During either of the first two steps, adjuvant medications (see chapter 6) are added if there is a specific pain condition that could benefit from them. Common indications for adjuvant medications may be neuropathic pain, visceral pain, or sympathetically mediated pain. There are less structured guidelines for using adjuvant medications. Most doctors simply start with the ones most likely to help and least likely to cause side effects, then try a series of them until good pain relief is achieved. Adjuvant medications often take several weeks to work, however, so it is important not to abandon a trial too soon.

There may be some variations in using the WHO steps depending on the cause and severity of the person's pain. For example, anti-inflammatory medications rarely, if ever, benefit neuropathic pain, so the first step may be skipped in patients with purely neuropathic pain. Some doctors recommend using antidepressants as adjuvants in every patient with significant pain, while others only use them in certain conditions.

The third step of the WHO ladder, invasive treatments and palliative therapy, are used when patients do not get adequate pain relief with anti-inflammatory and opioid medications. In recent years, however, many doctors have decided that palliative chemotherapy and radiation therapy should be used earlier and more frequently for pain control. This has led some to suggest that these two therapies should be considered the third step, with invasive therapies being assigned as a fourth step.

The first two steps, along with adjuvant medications, are considered enough to control "90 percent of the pain 90 percent of the time in 90 percent of patients." The 90 percent rule is often used as the deciding factor in attempting a more invasive or aggressive therapy; if a person has good pain control 90 percent of the time, he is considered successfully treated. Those who do not get that much relief are candidates for the more aggressive pain treatments summarized in the rest of this chapter.

Pain from Cancer Invasion into Bone

Bone invasion, or metastasis, is one of the most common causes of pain in cancer patients. Of all the patients who develop cancer, about 30 to 70 percent eventually develop metastases to one or more bones. Cancers of the breast, kidney, lung, and prostate are more likely to invade bones than are other types of cancer. The bones most commonly invaded are the vertebrae (spine), pelvis, and long bones of the arms or legs.

When treating cancer pain arising from bone, two different types of therapy are used at the same time. The first and most effective treatment is radiation, and sometimes chemotherapy, to kill the tumor cells. Radiation therapy is particularly effective for treating most forms of bone pain, sometimes relieving the pain in a matter of days. If the tumor can be completely destroyed, the bone may (or may not) heal completely, but further destruction of the bone will be stopped. In a few cases, the bone may continue to weaken even after the tumor is destroyed, however. Even when the tumor is not completely destroyed, significant pain relief is obtained in 70 to 80 percent of cases, with few side effects.

Patients who have several bony metastases in different locations may benefit from radiation given internally, rather than standard X-ray radiation. A radioactive chemical, strontium-89, that collects in the bones is used for this purpose. When it is given to patients with bone metastases, it concentrates at the area of metastasis, destroying the tumor. The therapy is almost as successful as external radiation, which is quite impressive when one considers that it is generally used in persons with widespread cancer. For example, several studies have reported strontium-89 gives 50 to 70 percent pain relief in patients with prostate cancer that has involved several bones. Strontium-89 can destroy some of the blood-forming cells of the bone marrow, so it should not be used in patients receiving other chemotherapy.

At the same time that radiation or chemotherapy is being planned, immediate efforts are made to treat the reaction and pain occurring within the bone. Treatments usually include medications such as opioids and anti-inflammatory medications taken by mouth. In some cases, particularly when the spinal bones are involved, injection of cortisone into the area provides immediate relief (see chapter 10). Cortisone taken by mouth can also be effective, although high doses may be required.

Some other medication can reduce the pain of bony metastasis by slowing the destruction of bone. Biphosphonate drugs, such as etidronate, clodronate, and pamidronate, slow the destruction of bone in some forms of cancer, reducing bone pain significantly. These drugs can all cause kidney and stomach problems that sometimes limit their usefulness, however. Calcitonin, a naturally occurring hormone, also slows the destruction of bone. It is available as a simple-to-use nasal spray, so it can be taken even by persons who cannot take oral medications. Implanted intrathecal pumps (see chapter 11) provide a final alternative that may be effective when other treatments do not work.

Finally, it's important to remember that simple mechanical therapies can reduce the pain from weakened bones considerably. Braces, slings, and other items that reduce movement of the affected area can dramatically reduce pain until other therapies have a chance to work. When the bones of the leg, pelvis, or lower back are involved, simply avoiding weight bearing by using a wheelchair or walker may help immensely.

Neuropathic Pain

Neuropathic pain (see chapters 1 and 2) is not caused by any actual damage to the tissues of the body. Instead, it is caused directly from damaged nerve tissue. The term *neuropathic pain* is generally used to mean that the nerve tissue is damaged internally. True neuropathic pain does not have a curable external cause. The terms *nerve compression* or *nerve entrapment* are used if the nerve is internally normal but is being compressed or stretched by tumor or scar tissue. These problems can often be cured by removing the compression or entrapment.

It is important to know that there is no test to show neuropathic pain. The damage is microscopic and cannot be seen on an MRI or CT scan. A scar or tumor entrapping or compressing a nerve may be seen on an MRI scan, however. A test called a nerve conduction study *may* show internal nerve damage when it is severe, but most physicians rely on the patient's description of her pain to make the diagnosis.

Neuropathic pain usually has characteristics that are described as a constant burning, often with sudden episodes (called paroxysms) of shooting pains or electrical shock sensations. The pain is often aggravated by movement or by touching or stimulating certain areas near the location of the pain. The area involved in neuropathic pain is usually quite sensitive compared to other areas of the body. Two different terms are used to describe the hypersensitivity. Hyperalgesia (pronounced "high-purr-all-gees-yah") is a severe pain caused by what should be a mildly painful stimulus, such as deep pressure or light scraping. Allodynia (pronounced "al-oh-din-ee-ah") is the sensation of pain caused by a normally nonpainful stimulus, such as light touch.

Neuropathic pain is caused by several mechanisms. Damaged but still living nerve fibers often send out abnormal signals that are interpreted as pain by the brain. In some cases, the absence of normal signals (as could occur when the nerve fibers are completely destroyed) is also interpreted as painful by the brain. There may also be "short circuiting" between nerve fibers, so that what should be sensed as a temperature change, for example, is actually sensed as pain.

The primary treatment of neuropathic pain involves using the adjunctive medications such as antidepressants, antiseizure medications, and benzodiazepines to stop the damaged nerve fibers from sending out abnormal messages (see chapter 6). It is important to remember these treatments are not like taking a pain pill; you do not get relief half an hour after you take the medicine. Rather adjuvant medications are more like chemotherapy. If you continue to take the medications for several weeks, you will begin to see results. As mentioned earlier, treatment with opioid (narcotic) or anti-inflammatory medications is usually not very effective against neuropathic pain.

Neurostimulation (see chapter 10) is often beneficial, however, and should be tried if medications are not effective.

Neuromas

Neuromas are actually a type of neuropathic pain, since they are caused by abnormalities within the nerve itself. They differ a bit from most kinds of neuropathic pain, however, because they occur after direct damage to a nerve, such as might happen during surgery. After a nerve is severed, it tries to grow back to the tissue it should serve. If this growth cannot occur properly, a neuroma may form. The neuroma is an abnormal growth of nerve fibers and scar tissue that appears as a swelling or ball on the nerve.

Some neuromas are very painful, while others cause no discomfort. Several factors may account for this variation. Small, hard neuromas that consist mostly of scar tissue with few nerve fibers are often not painful. Larger, soft neuromas containing a large number of regenerating nerve fibers are usually very painful. The location of the neuroma may also be important. Neuromas in parts of the body subjected to movement and external pressure are likely to be irritated more often than those in less sensitive locations.

Neuroma pain usually begins days or weeks after a surgical procedure. The pain is similar to that experienced from other kinds of neuropathic pain, but usually only involves the area of one peripheral nerve. Most patients can find a single trigger area that causes severe shooting pain if they press on it or tap over it. The trigger area is usually directly over the neuroma.

Neuroma pain may respond to the same treatments used for other neuropathic pains, but because it occurs in a single location, other therapies may be used. Injecting local anesthetic and cortisone into the area of the neuroma is often very helpful. Physical therapy using stretching, ultrasound, and vibration may also be effective, but its success varies greatly. In many cases, neuroma pain will slowly go away over several months, no matter what therapy is used.

If the location of the neuroma is known exactly, surgical removal of the neuroma may stop the pain. Simply exploring an old incision in hopes of finding and removing a neuroma is almost never successful, however. It is almost impossible to dissect a tiny nerve out of the scar tissue left from previous surgery. If the location of the neuroma is not known exactly and medications are ineffective, neurostimulation is usually a more effective option than attempting to find the neuroma surgically.

Specific Neuropathic Pain Syndromes

Neuropathic pain can be caused by almost every kind of tumor and several types of therapy. It can occur in almost any part of the body. However, several syndromes (a group of related symptoms seen together in people who have a similar condition) are commonly seen in cancer patients. Many of these syndromes occur only in patients who have had surgery. Although the reasons for this are not entirely clear, obviously surgery will directly damage or cut some small nerves, while the surgical scars may compress others.

The combination of surgery with radiation or chemotherapy appears to make the development of a neuropathic pain syndrome more likely.

Tumor Infiltration Near a Nerve

Tumors pressing on or growing into nerve tissue are a frequent cause of neuropathic pain in cancer patients. This can occur almost anywhere in the body, but common locations involve the nerves going to the leg (cancers of the rectum and gynecologic organs) or the arm (cancer of the upper lobe of the lung). The pain that occurs is usually both aching and burning, often radiating into the involved limb. Shooting or shocking pains are less common with tumor infiltration near a nerve than with other causes of neuropathic pain. On the other hand, weakness in the involved area occurs more often with tumor compression than with other types of neuropathic pain. Swelling of the affected limb is often significant. The first step in treatment is to relieve the compression with radiation or chemotherapy. Otherwise, the treatment is similar to that for other forms of neuropathic pain.

Postradiation Neuropathy

Radiation can cause peripheral nerve injury, probably not by damaging the actual nerve fibers, but rather by creating microscopic scars within the nerve that irritate the fibers. The resultant neuropathic pain usually appears months or years following radiation treatment. The strongest hint that the pain is caused by postradiation neuropathy is the location: It usually involves only the area that received radiation. Compared to the pain caused by tumor compression, postradiation pain is generally less severe, has less aching but more burning characteristics, and progresses more slowly. Weakness is unusual in postradiation neuropathy, although abnormal sensations may occur. Swelling is usually not severe, if it occurs at all.

The treatment of postradiation neuropathy is usually done entirely with medications. In the last several years, pain clinics have begun using certain specially made ointments that absorb through the skin. These ointments are placed right at the site of pain, delivering the medications directly to the damaged nerves. This may be more effective for postradiation neuropathy than oral medications and may cause fewer side effects.

Postchemotherapy Neuropathy

Chemotherapy tends to cause a peripheral neuropathy, since the longest nerve fibers (the ones going to fingers and toes) are affected the most. Chemotherapy-induced neuropathy usually begins during the course of chemotherapy and may improve after the therapy is completed. Certain types of chemotherapy medications are more likely to cause this problem than are others. (See the list in chapter 3.)

Postchemotherapy neuropathy usually begins with numbness and burning pain involving the feet and to a lesser extent the fingertips. Unlike most other forms of neuropathic pain, this pain usually involves both sides of the body equally. In addition to the burning pain, hyperalgesia and allodynia (see page 212) are common. Leg cramps and mild leg weakness may be felt. Some patients develop symptoms similar to those of sympathetically mediated pain (discussed below), especially those who have undergone therapy with vincristine, cisplatin, or paclitaxel.

Medications are usually effective in reducing the pain, and the symptoms may stop entirely a few weeks or months after the chemotherapy is completed. For a few people, however, the neuropathic pain continues permanently. Neurostimulation (see chapter 11) can be effective if the painful area is not too large. If both the hands and the feet are involved, neurostimulation may require inserting two separate electrodes, however.

Postoperative Syndromes

Although the locations of postoperative pain syndromes differ, the treatment is the same in almost every case. The standard adjunctive medications are always used, often with benzodiazepines or antispasmodics (see chapter 6) added to relieve muscle spasms. High doses of cortisone are sometimes effective if begun when the symptoms first appear, but usually are not effective later.

Physical therapy is often very helpful since most of these syndromes involve damage to the muscles as well as the nerves. The therapy should focus on stretching the muscles and restoring strength, however, not just treatments like hot packs or massage. Nerve blocks (see chapter 10) are often a mainstay of treatment for all these conditions. Neurostimulation (see chapter 11) may be helpful, particularly in controlling the burning pain, but usually does not relieve the syndrome by itself.

Post–Radical Neck Dissection Syndrome

This occurs only in a few patients who have had a radical neck dissection for cancers of the throat and mouth. The syndrome may begin soon after surgery and is much more common in patients who received radiation treatment to shrink the tumor before surgery. Most persons affected complain of tightness, a burning sensation, and numbness involving the neck and shoulder on the side of the dissection. There may also be weakness of the shoulder muscle on the affected side.

Postmastectomy Syndrome

This condition occurs in up to 5 percent of women following a mastectomy. It is also more common in those who have had radiation therapy to the area. The pain is usually described as a burning sensation in the armpit, back of the arm, and chest wall. There is usually a tight sensation that makes moving the shoulder difficult, and movement of the arm tends to make the pain worse. Swelling of the arm often occurs and is made worse by the lack of movement. The condition may begin a few days after surgery or not until weeks later.

Medications can be helpful, but the most important treatment for postmastectomy syndrome is an aggressive physical therapy program that restores movement and motion. This not only relieves pain (eventually); it will reduce swelling and prevent the condition from becoming worse. The therapy can be quite painful at first, however, so it is important that medications to relieve the pain are given before therapy is started. Nerve blocks can also be very helpful, especially if there is a trigger area in the scar or chest wall that causes radiating pain.

Postthoracotomy Syndrome

This condition follows a thoracotomy—a surgical incision made between the ribs to enter the chest, usually for surgery to remove lung cancer. The pain is usually limited to the side of the chest, usually below the incision. Aching and burning pain radiate along one or two ribs to the front of the chest. There is usually no loss of sensation, although sometimes an area on the front of the abdomen may feel numb. The skin may be hypersensitive.

In many cases, an area in the scar or near the small puncture scars from the chest tubes is exquisitely tender. Pressure over the tender point causes the pain to shoot around the chest wall. In such cases, nerve blocks are often very helpful. If they do not give long-term relief, a neurodestructive block may be tried (see chapter 10), or surgery to remove the painful area (which is usually a neuroma) can be attempted. If there is no trigger point, neurostimulation may be the most effective treatment.

Postnephrectomy Syndrome

Postnephrectomy syndrome sometimes follows the removal of a kidney. It is very similar to postthoracotomy pain, although it occurs lower on the flank, rather than on the chest wall. There may be numbness or a heavy sensation in the flank, and the pain sometimes radiates into the groin. Unfortunately, therapy for postnephrectomy pain is not as successful as that for postthoracotomy syndrome. Nerve blocks and neurostimulation are sometimes effective, however.

Sympathetically Mediated Pain (Complex Regional Pain Syndrome)

Sympathetic pain was first described in 1864 as a syndrome of severe burning pain seen in some Civil War soldiers after nerve injury. The primary symptom of sympathetic pain is severe, burning pain and extreme hypersensitivity in the affected area. Light touch, temperature changes, and movement may all increase the pain. Edema (swelling) is usually present. Temperature changes (the skin becomes either warm or cool), abnormal sweating of the area, and abnormal coloration (either bluish or red) of the skin are sometimes experienced.

Sympathetically mediated pain involves the sympathetic nervous system (the unconscious part of the nervous system controlling functions like sweating and blood flow). The problem is quite complex and poorly understood, however. It is now apparent that not only sympathetic nerves, but also regular sensory nerves and abnormal levels of many neuronal chemicals are all involved in the condition. The condition may begin after any type of nerve damage that causes neuropathic pain, or after a pathologic fracture that occurs when tumor invades bones. It is more common if the damage involves the foot or the hand, but it has occurred in almost every part of the body.

When sympathetic pain does occur, it must be treated immediately and aggressively. If it is not successfully treated within a few months, it usually worsens and may even spread into areas where no nerve damage has occurred. The affected area becomes atrophied (wasted) and the joints lose mobility. Once the area has become wasted, the chance for recovery is bleak. In such cases, the pain may worsen, although not always. Because of the risk that sympathetically mediated pain may worsen and become permanent, it is the one type of pain for which a pain specialist should be consulted immediately.

No single therapy is effective in all cases, so an aggressive, multiple therapy approach is used. The treatment usually includes medications, active physical therapy, and sympathetic nerve blocks. Opioid medications are required for pain relief, and some other medications, including tricyclic antidepressants and antiseizure medications, may be helpful. Cortisone and medications that block the sympathetic nerves, such as clonidine, may also be tried.

Nerve blocks of the sympathetic nerves are very effective in some cases, but completely ineffective in others. Surgical sympathectomy (cutting the sympathetic nerves) to the affected area may be performed if nerve blocks give only temporary relief, but is not helpful if the nerve blocks give no relief at all. Surgical implantation of a neurostimulator may provide significant pain relief if other therapies are not effective.

Physical therapy to maintain or improve joint motion and desensitize the affected area is always a mainstay of treatment for sympathetic pain. A few reported cases claim that physical therapy alone may be sufficient to stop the disease if it is started early. Most patients, however, find therapy extremely painful. A team approach using nerve blocks and medications to provide pain relief so that the patient can tolerate an aggressive physical therapy program is generally thought to give the best results.

Visceral Pain

Visceral pain (see chapter 1 for a more detailed discussion) is usually caused by two conditions in cancer patients: obstruction or tumor invasion. Obstruction pain involves a partial obstruction of the bowel or a duct that carries fluid from one organ to another. This type of pain can, of course, be caused by a tumor compressing the hollow organ. It can also be caused by surgical or radiation scarring that has thickened and shortened over time (as most scars do), causing partial obstruction of the duct. The pain of obstruction is usually cramping or colicky in nature and often waxes and wanes in severity.

When tumor causes the obstruction, radiation, chemotherapy, or surgery, depending on which is most appropriate for the problem, may relieve the obstruction. In a few cases, corticosteroids (cortisone) may be given to reduce swelling around the tumor in hopes of relieving the obstruction. If the obstruction is caused by scarring, the best solution is to surgically remove the scar. In an area that has had previous surgery or heavy irradiation, surgery is fairly risky and complicated, however. If the obstructive symptoms can be relieved by medications, it may be best to avoid surgery as long as possible.

A different type of visceral pain is caused by a tumor invading the internal organs or the wall of the abdomen. This pain is often described as aching or "boring," as though something is drilling through the back of the abdomen. This type of visceral pain often responds to opioid medications, but is not improved very much by the adjunctive medications. An implanted spinal infusion catheter may give better relief in such cases than oral or injected medications. Alternatively, a celiac plexus block (see chapter 10) can be tried, and if it relieves the pain, destruction of the plexus can be performed.

When the Cancer Is Cured, but the Pain Remains

It is important to realize, as you probably already have, that even when cancer treatment successfully destroys the tumor and the patient has been "cured," there may have been significant damage to the body. In fact, some patients in this situation find themselves almost every bit as anxious and depressed as they were when they had cancer. Often, family members and even the cancer physician do not seem to understand why they still have pain. Some people in this situation worry that they are just addicted to the pain medication and cannot stop taking it.

The reality is that as many as 15 percent of cancer patients who are completely cured of their cancers still have significant pain problems.

Most have neuropathic pain, although some are left with visceral pain. Pain is more likely in patients who have had major surgical procedures as part of their cancer treatments, in those who have had radiation near major nerves or the pelvis, and in those who have had certain chemotherapies associated with nerve damage.

Unfortunately, in many of these cases, the cause of the pain does not get better as time goes on. However, the same treatments that are effective in people while they have cancer are just as effective (if not more so) in those who have been cured of cancer. Often, the oncologist is not willing to continue refilling all those medications. He is focused on treating cancer, not pain in people who no longer have cancer. Your family doctor may be willing to take on the task, but if not, you can ask for a referral to a physician who primarily treats pain.

CHAPTER 13

Participating in Experimental Medical Trials

by Roger S. Cicala, M.D.

A Word of Caution About Research

Medical research is many things. Of course, it is one of the primary ways of advancing medical science. It's not the only way medicine makes progress, though. A lot of the advances in medicine do not come from carefully directed scientific research. They may come from insights and observations made in everyday clinical practice, from unrelated research in basic sciences that have a medical application, and sometimes by investigating "folk wisdom" and "old wives' remedies."

Every new medication and treatment must undergo a period of controlled medical research before it can be prescribed by doctors in practice for use by the public, however. This research is not what most people think of as research. There is no medical scientist alone in the lab who suddenly shouts "Eureka!" and releases a newly discovered medication for the betterment of humanity. Rather, huge teams of scientists, usually working in industrial or university laboratories, carefully design or isolate substances that may be useful as medicines. Each substance is tested in animals, usually for years, to determine its safety and possible uses. A few such substances undergo very limited trials in humans. Of those substances, probably fewer than one in a hundred ever becomes a useful medical treatment. For those that do, the process often takes ten years or more.

In addition to advancing medical science, research is a multibillion-dollar industry. Every pharmaceutical company is trying desperately to find the next billion-dollar-a-year drug, knowing that only a tiny fraction of the drugs they test will ever make it to market. A huge government bureaucracy does its own research and parcels out multimillion-dollar grants to academic scientists who do more research. There are large companies whose only function is to perform clinical trials for drug companies and the government. Other companies and consultants advise scientists in how to obtain government grants for research and how to make profits doing clinical trials for pharmaceutical companies.

This does not mean that medical research is bad or entirely mercenary. On the contrary, it is why the medical field has advanced further than almost any other area of science in this century. However, many people think that a new drug currently under research is probably better than what is already available on the market. This is sometimes true, but one must remember that most drugs undergoing clinical trials will never even be proven good enough to be marketed. Others will be found too dangerous to use.

Most of the people involved in research are very altruistic. I know dozens of doctors who work for a fraction of what they could make in private practice just because they want to do research. The motives of some people involved in research are not always altruistic, however. Marketing and businesspeople, not to mention physicians, all realize that most of the public considers a research center to be a bit better than a regular hospital or clinic. A lot of people use the label of "research" to sell products and treatments. Others are doing research largely because they can make money at it or advance their careers.

Cancer patients, in particular, are often desperate for something new and miraculous that may cure their disease. Those who have been told their disease is terminal feel they have nothing to lose and that they should try anything. This may be true, and I encourage anyone in that position to try any experimental treatment that has even the slightest chance of helping.

What a person should *not* do is abandon accepted medical treatments because a newer treatment is available in a research study, even if "preliminary" results indicate the research treatment is better. Remember that most new treatments show their best results when the numbers are derived from a few (in research, a few may mean several thousand) carefully monitored and treated cases. The results when a treatment enters general use are rarely as good. There are dozens of horror stories about just such situations.

For example, some years ago a trial for a new combination chemotherapy regimen for breast cancer was begun. One of the researchers was so excited about the excellent preliminary results of the study that he inappropriately released the results to a newspaper. Thousands of people demanded access to the treatment, even going so far as to sue their insurance companies to force them to pay for the treatment. Special circumstances were declared because of the public pressure, and patients were allowed to take the experimental treatment instead of the routine treatments being used. Two years later, it was determined that the experimental treatment was not nearly as successful as the routine treatment. In short, the people who took the experimental treatment were much *less* likely to be cured than those who had standard therapy. The preliminary results were just that—preliminary.

Researchers are people, too, and some of them are not honest. In the 1980s, breast cancer treatment was completely changed when a large study showed a simple lumpectomy and radiation was just as likely to provide a cure as a complete mastectomy. Ten years later, after hundreds of thousands of women with breast cancer had a lumpectomy, it was revealed that the original researcher had falsified the data and done improper statistical analysis of the results. For many patients, lumpectomy reduced the chance of cure.

At any rate, our purpose is not to scare you away from participating in a research study that may help you. It is simply to make certain that you know the odds before participating in such a trial. A given experimental treatment may be as good or better than what is available to the public. Just because it is new and experimental, however, does not mean that it is better.

What Is a Clinical Trial?

A clinical trial is an organized study conducted to answer specific questions about a new treatment or a new way of using a known treatment. In most cases, clinical trials compare the best-known standard therapy with a newer therapy to see if one produces more cures or causes fewer side effects than the other does. Other types of studies evaluate the quality of life in cancer patients or evaluate cancer prevention therapies. A trial may involve new anticancer drugs, new combinations of drugs already in use, or new ways of administering a treatment. Depending on what is being studied, a particular clinical trial may involve patients with cancer or people who do not have cancer but who are at higher risk than most people for developing it.

Before a treatment is made available for clinical trial, it is carefully studied in laboratory animals. After that, it is allowed to be used in small, carefully controlled clinical trials in people. Clinical trials proceed in an organized series of steps, each with its own rules and regulations. Each step is identified as a certain phase of trial. The first phases simply test a drug for safety and dosage. Later phases focus on the benefit of the therapy. Cancer clinical trials usually fall into one of three phases.

Phase I trials are the first studies of a new treatment done in humans. They are used to determine the safety and safe dosage range of a drug and to evaluate how the drug should be administered (orally, by injection, etc.) and how often it should be given. A Phase I trial involves only a small number of patients, often studied one or two at a time. Small doses are given at first and then increased until side effects begin to develop.

Phase I trials are generally only offered to cancer patients whose tumor cannot be helped by any known treatment. They do not determine if a treatment is effective or not, only if it is safe. Since the participants are not expected to benefit from the medication, these trials usually pay a stipend to persons willing to enroll in the study.

Phase II trials are designed to provide preliminary information about the effectiveness of the treatment. They do not determine if the treatment is better than other treatments, only if it may be effective. Each Phase II study focuses on a particular type of cancer. The study is usually considered successful if 20 percent or more of the participants show shrinking of their tumors.

In most cases, only patients with tumors that are not responsive to standard therapies are eligible to participate in Phase II trials. These studies involve more study subjects (usually twenty-five to fifty persons) than Phase I trials, but only a few centers participate so that the study can be very closely monitored. Because more people participate in Phase II trials than were involved in the Phase I study, some side effects of the treatment may not become apparent until this phase of study.

Phase III trials compare a treatment that has been successful in Phase II trials to the accepted treatment for a certain type of cancer. The trial may evaluate a promising new drug, combination of drugs, or procedure, comparing it with the current standard treatment. Phase III studies are large, consisting of hundreds or even thousands of patients studied in a dozen or more different cancer centers and clinics nationwide.

Patients participating in a Phase III study are randomized; some receive the new treatment while others receive the standard treatment. In most cases, the study is also blinded (patients do not know what treatment they receive) or double-blinded (neither the patients nor the doctor know which treatment they receive) until after the study is over. Blinding is done to eliminate any placebo effect or investigator bias about the new treatment. If you are assigned the standard treatment, you receive what experts view as the best treatment available in current routine medical practice. If you are assigned the new treatment, you receive a treatment that some experts think may have significant advantages over the standard. The reason the clinical trial has been initiated is that the superiority of one treatment over the other has not yet been firmly established.

Some treatments enter a fourth phase called Group C. These are usually drugs or treatments awaiting FDA approval that are available for certain doctors or treatment centers (usually ones who performed the Phase III studies) to continue to use and collect further data. The term "Phase IV trial" describes any continuing evaluation that takes place after FDA approval, when the drug is already on the market and available for general use (postmarketing surveillance).

Some supportive care, prevention, and screening trials are not done in phases, but instead simply compare groups of people using a certain anticancer strategy (counseling, behavior change, detection method) with those who do not. In this type of study, there is no medical risk, so FDA control is less stringent.

Protocols, Eligibility, and Randomization

Clinical trials follow strict scientific guidelines written as a protocol before the study begins. The protocol includes the study's design, who can participate, what tests and treatments will be done during the study, and what information will be gathered. It also determines how many people will be enrolled in the study, what drugs the participants will take as part of the study, and what treatments they may have outside the study. Every doctor and center that participates in the study uses the same protocol so that information from all the centers can be combined and compared.

The trial may only involve participants at one or two highly specialized centers, or it may take place at dozens of hospitals and clinics at the same time. At each location, a physician is designated as the study director. Other physicians, nurses, and pharmacists may work with the study director, but all are under her supervision. A national study director oversees the activities of all the centers involved and coordinates the gathering and sharing of information from all of the sites. No matter which site a patient is seen at, the study protocol assures that all patients at all sites receive exactly the same treatment and follow the same rules.

Because the study wants to investigate only the study treatment, the protocol tries to keep every other factor (called a variable in study jargon) identical for every patient. The protocol identifies, as strictly as possible, the characteristics that participants must have. These eligibility criteria usually include age, gender, the type of cancer a person has, how far the cancer has progressed, other treatments the patient has had in the past, other medical conditions he may have, and many other factors.

Eligibility criteria are extremely important parts of the protocol, assuring that the study results are not influenced by outside factors. They are also needed to help identify which type of patient is most likely to benefit from the treatment in question. For example, a new drug may work for people with an early stage of cancer, but not be effective in a later stage. In this situation, the protocol may require not allowing persons into the study if their cancer is too advanced. Eligibility criteria also help ensure patient safety by preventing people with known risks from participating. For example, some drugs can only be given safely if a person has normal kidney function.

Eligibility criteria cannot be waived for any individual. It is common for a person who wanted to participate in a study, but was turned down, to demand an exception be made. Scientifically, even a few exceptions could invalidate the results from an entire study. For this reason, the site director (the physician in charge of the study sites) does not have the authority to make an exception. In some cases, the protocol states that even the national director cannot make an exception.

As mentioned earlier, clinical trials are often randomized trials. This means some people will receive the drug or treatment that is being studied, while others will receive a standard treatment. No one can make sure you are placed in the group receiving the study treatment, since the trials are blinded. The actual drug or treatment you received will not be known until after the study is over, when a locked code is opened to identify the treatments.

Randomized, blinded studies are often used for things such as chemotherapy or other treatments that you only do once. (In the case of chemotherapy, it may be several medications given together, but medically it is considered one series of treatments.) If you participate in a blinded study, you usually have to agree not to change treatments or get additional treatment for the duration of the study. The physicians who monitor you during the study will take good medical care of you, though. If they determine, for example, that the treatment being studied is clearly not working for you, they will take you out of the study and make sure that you get other treatment.

Not all trials have completely randomized treatment, however. In some studies, known as crossover trials, each person receives the study drug for a certain amount of time, then another drug for a certain amount of time. The crossover may be blinded (that is, you do not know which medicine is which), but each person will receive each treatment at different times. Crossover trials are often used to study pain medications or other medicines that are used to control symptoms. Often, after you have tried each drug in such a study, you get to choose which one you would like to continue for a longer, follow-up period.

How Are Research Participants Protected?

Clinical trials have several procedures to protect the safety of the people who participate. The organization that sponsors the study (for example, the National Cancer Institute) will have approved the protocol involved. It also will have gotten approval from one or more outside review groups that were not part of their organization. Additionally, each study site will have the protocol reviewed and approved by an Institutional Review Board (IRB) that oversees clinical research at that facility. The board includes doctors, scientists, and sometimes medical ethicists or clergy. The IRB members do not have any personal interest in the study, but rather serve as neutral reviewers who make sure that no one who participates is likely to be harmed.

Finally, any Phase III trial is constantly monitored by an oversight group called a Data Safety and Monitoring Committee. This committee periodically monitors the safety of the participants and evaluates the early data to make sure that the study should continue as planned. If the Data Safety and Monitoring Committee ever decides there is any danger involved in the study, they can immediately stop it.

Before entering any trial, you will receive complete information about the study, so that you can give informed consent to participate. Informed consent means that you are given all the facts about a study before you decide whether to take part. This includes details about the treatments and tests you will receive and the possible benefits and risks they may have. After receiving all this information, you will be asked to sign a consent form. The form does not waive any of your rights; it simply means that you understood the rules, risks, and possible benefits of the study.

While you are actually participating in a study, you have a number of rights and protections. If, during the study, the investigators become aware of any new or additional risks of the study, they are required to inform you immediately. You may be asked to sign a new consent form if you want to stay in the study. If, at any time, you or the monitors believe that the treatment harms you, you will be taken off the study immediately. In fact, you have the right to leave a study at any time. The study coordinator can ask you to fill out a form stating your reasons for leaving and if you had any unpleasant effects from the study, but cannot penalize you in any way.

Why Participate in a Trial?

There are many advantages to participating in a controlled clinical trial of an experimental treatment. For patients who have been told there is no other hope, a trial may provide the only possibility of remission or cure. For others, a clinical trial may provide them access to an effective drug they could not receive otherwise. Clinical trials usually provide free care and often provide more intensive monitoring than an insurance company would be willing to pay for. Some trials even pay a small stipend for participating, or provide travel expenses when needed.

In many cases, the advantages do not end when the trial is over. Participants in trials often receive free follow-up care and much closer monitoring than they would otherwise receive, often for several years after the study is completed. Trials of pain medications sometimes continue to supply study participants with pain medications for a year or two after the study is over. In addition, participating as a subject in research may also benefit other people who later develop the same disease by finding a better treatment.

When you take part in a clinical trial, you receive your treatment in a cancer center, hospital, or clinic that is one of the study sites. The treatment team will follow your progress closely. In fact, you probably will have more tests and doctor visits than you would if you were not taking part in a study. You will have to follow the treatment plan outlined by the study protocol, and you may have other responsibilities, such as keeping a log or filling out forms about your health. You can continue to see your own doctor whenever you wish, but you must notify the study team of any treatments he prescribes.

Participating in clinical trials is an individual decision. There are definite benefits for some people, while others may only inconvenience themselves by participating. On the other hand, there can be real risks involved. Some treatments that initially appear effective are later found not to be as effective as the standard therapy; others are found to have long-lasting side effects that were not discovered until after the trial was finished.

How to Find Out About
Legitimate Clinical Trials

The largest number of legitimate research studies are coordinated through the National Cancer Institute (NCI). More than forty-five research-oriented institutions have been designated by the National Cancer Institute as Clinical Cancer Centers. Located throughout the country, they play an important role in cancer research. All these institutes have met certain standards of the NCI and are allowed to coordinate research studies and evaluate new technologies. The NCI has also organized the Cooperative Clinical Trials Program, which joins researchers, cancer centers, and community physicians into a number of groups that conduct clinical trials. These cooperative groups place approximately twenty thousand new patients into large, Phase III trials each year.

The NCI also has organized the Community Clinical Oncology Program (CCOP). This program links community physicians with research teams in cancer centers, allowing clinical trials to enroll patients from smaller communities. This enables doctors to offer patients the opportunity to participate in clinical trials without having to travel long distances or leave their usual caregivers. Several of these programs focus on encouraging minority populations to participate in trials.

If you are interested in finding out about NCI-directed studies that are available, the institute has created a computer file about cancer clinical trials called the Physicians Data Query (PDQ). The information in PDQ is updated monthly to show the latest clinical trials being offered around the country. Patients can obtain PDQ information by contacting the Cancer Information Service (see Appendix F for the Internet address).

Many studies do not take place directly under the auspices of the National Cancer Institute. These are often studies organized by pharmaceutical companies or companies that manufacture medical devices, to demonstrate that their products are safe and effective. Such studies are required before the Food and Drug Administration (FDA) will permit companies to sell and advertise the drug or device. Other studies are started by individual physician investigators at cancer centers and other health care institutions. Appendix F lists many of the major cancer investigation sites in the United States.

Making Sure a Trial Is Truly Research

As mentioned earlier, some studies involve individual clinics or small groups of physicians. Unfortunately, some rather unscrupulous persons use the word *research* simply to attract patients into their facility or practice. Some of these people mean well and may actually think they offer a better way of doing things. Many of them, however, are medical con artists preying on desperate people. Although participating in such a "study" probably will not hurt you physically, it can be devastating emotionally and financially.

In more than a few cases, patients have been told insurance will cover their participation in such a study, only to find out months later it did not and that they are responsible for the bills. Even more disgusting, in a few cases such con artists never billed the patients while they were alive, and then sent large "medical" bills to their estates, assuming that no one would question the bills at that time.

At the very least, a real clinical trial will usually provide you with free medication. If you are asked to pay for your medication or to pay a fee to participate in a study, you should question whether it is a legitimate study. If you are told your health insurance will cover an experimental medication, you should contact your insurer directly. Health insurance plans do not cover experimental treatments or medications that are not approved for general use.

If you have any doubts about the legitimacy of a study, there are several questions you should ask. Find out what institution is directing the study. Most studies are conducted by university medical centers or well-known regional hospitals. Small clinics and private practices occasionally participate in legitimate studies, but are rarely the center of such a study. Rather, they should be able to tell you clearly where the study center is located and who monitors the study. Usually, there will be a coordinating center that is part of an academic institution, or a major drug company will be funding and monitoring the study.

If the funding is coming from a drug company whose name you recognize, then it is almost certainly legitimate. If you do not know the name, ask to see the documentation that the study is supervised by the FDA. If the FDA is not supervising the study, chances are very small that the study is legitimate. No treatment will ever be approved for general use without an FDA-sanctioned study. Some small, pilot studies do take place without FDA supervision, but you should seriously question whether you want to participate in such a study.

There are several catchwords and jargon terms frequently associated with fly-by-night operations. "All natural," "herbal," or "completely safe" are not medical terms, they are marketing terms. They also mean "These substances are not really medications, therefore they are not regulated by the government, so I can do whatever I want with them." There are certainly lots of safe and effective herbal or natural products (chapter 9 discusses many), but they should not be thought of as newly researched treatments. I can clip grass out of my backyard and market it as an herbal cancer cure. No one can stop me until they have scientifically proven I am a fraud, which could take several years.

Another favorite catchword is "secret," especially in "ancient secret" or "secret Oriental cure." Trust us, if there were a secret cure for cancer out there, someone would have marketed it and gotten the billions of dollars that would result. For the same reason, there are no government agency or drug company plots to keep a cancer cure secret. There would simply be too much potential profit in such a treatment for any organization to keep it suppressed.

Finally, the Internet has become a wonderful tool for both learning about your particular disease and contacting others for support and information. Always remember, though, that the Internet is not edited and not subject to review by professional or medical organizations. People can put up very professional-looking Internet sites and say anything they please, which may or may not be based on facts. Unfortunately, more than a few doctors have "research" sites that actually offer nothing more than a routine consultation, for which the doctor will send a bill. (I found twenty-three sites that clearly did this during a recent Internet search for prostate cancer.) Legitimate research studies never bill patients for evaluating them as study candidates.

CHAPTER 14

Hospice Care

by Daniel Brookoff, M.D.

It was not very long ago that people with advanced cancer were left to suffer in pain and loneliness by health caregivers who felt that they had nothing left to offer. The philosophy of hospice is that for certain people with cancer or other diseases, a point can be reached where medical therapy no longer offers any realistic hope for cure or recovery. However, there are still days to be spent in this life, and those days are precious. Hospice care is an intense form of care focused on the relief of symptoms and on getting the most out of the life that remains.

Although many people think the function of hospice is to help people die, hospice is really there to help people live as free from pain and symptoms as possible while maintaining family ties and personal dignity. Its focus is on comfort and family, which is a radical departure for traditional medical care.

Hospice care is actually a return to earlier days of medical care when the physician's motto was "To cure sometimes, to relieve often, to comfort always." With hospice care, patients in the advanced stages of cancer can find relief and comfort. Both the patient and her family can take the time to become mentally and spiritually prepared for death. From a practical standpoint, hospice care provides the highest levels of pain relief and comfort in an environment that is far less invasive and intrusive than a hospital. It allows the patient to decide what he does or does not want during the end of life.

The History of Hospice

The history of the hospice movement is older than the history of medicine itself. In ancient Greece, there were healing temples where the dying were given special physical and emotional care. This type of care was practiced in many other ancient cultures. For example, in ancient Mayan temples, special foods and medicinal herbs were reserved solely for the dying. In the Middle Ages, taking time to care for the dying was seen as a religious duty of Crusading nobles. Many groups of Crusaders, such as the Knights of Malta, were originally founded as nursing orders.

Nursing care remained largely the province of the religious orders in Western culture until the mid-nineteenth century, when Florence Nightingale introduced the concept of the professional nurse. With the advent of hospitals in the late nineteenth century, medical and nursing care became more focused on the application of technology and less centered on comforting and caring. Death became institutionalized. Families were eventually separated from their dying loved ones, who could no longer die at home but spent their last days in hospitals or nursing homes. Death progressed from being a natural and accepted part of life to being a hidden event. At the same time, early misconceptions led many people to believe that all diseases were contagious. Fear of associating with the dying further separated cancer patients from their families, friends, and associates. People with advanced cancer were often left to spend many of their last hours alone.

The modern hospice movement began in 1842 with the founding of hospices in Lyons, France, by Jeanne Garnier. The Irish Sisters of Charity opened hospices in Dublin and London around the turn of the century. The first hospice in the United States, Calvary Hospital, opened in New York City in 1899, modeled on the works of the Sisters of Charity. It continues to operate to this day.

In 1967, Dame Cicely Saunders opened St. Christopher's Hospice in England. She set down the principles for hospice care that are still followed today:

- Emphasizing symptom control.
- Providing interdisciplinary care, not just medical care.

• Involving volunteers in the caring process.

• Caring for the patient and the family as a unit.

• Providing follow-up care for family members after a patient's death.

Interest in the dying process in the United States soared in 1969 with the publication of a book by Dr. Elizabeth Kübler-Ross, *On Death and Dying*, which broke new ground by discussing the way the dying were abandoned by their caregivers and separated from their families. This inspired resurgence of the American hospice movement in 1974, when the Hospice of Connecticut was started as a home-based hospice care organization funded by a three-year grant from the National Cancer Institute. In 1978, the National Hospice Organization was formed to promote the principles and philosophy of hospice care.

Despite the fact that hospice care has existed for so long, most Americans date the beginning of hospice care in the United States to 1982, when Medicare began to provide financial reimbursement for hospice care. Since that time, many American hospice services have been molded around the Medicare regulations and have adopted them as part of their core philosophies. Following the lead of Medicare, most private health insurance plans now provide coverage for hospice care. Medicaid currently covers hospice care in forty-three states and in the District of Columbia.

Who Is Eligible for Hospice Care?

As of 1999, there were more than three thousand active hospice programs in the United States caring for more than half a million patients. More than two hundred and twenty thousand Medicare beneficiaries receive hospice care each year. Eighty percent of those are diagnosed with cancer. Although the overwhelming majority of patients admitted to hospice care do have cancer, anyone with a terminal illness is eligible.

There are three general or philosophical criteria for admission of terminally ill patients to a hospice:

1. The patient has completed all active treatment to cure the disease.
2. The patient understands the diagnosis and prognosis.
3. The patient and family understand the goals of hospice care.

There are other standard criteria for admission to a hospice based on the regulations regarding Medicare hospice benefits, namely that the person has approximately six months or less left to live. Obviously, predicting mortality with this accuracy is beyond the abilities of medical science, and estimates of life expectancy are, at best, educated guesses. In a recent study, for example, the median survival after enrollment in a hospice was thirty-six days. However, 15 percent of hospice patients died within a week of enrollment, while 15 percent lived longer than six months.

Despite the fact that no one can make accurate predictions of how long a person may live, particularly since many patients thrive during hospice care, insurance companies always insist on some criteria for such things. The current guidelines that must be met to admit a person to hospice care include the generic criteria listed above, plus some medical criteria that may vary slightly depending on the geographic area and the health insurance plan involved. Following is a list of generally accepted guidelines for hospice admission. They may seem unnecessarily complex (probably because they are), but the simple fact is that almost any terminal cancer patient who wishes to receive hospice care is qualified to do so.

1. The patient is terminally ill and has been informed of this by his or her physician ("terminally ill" is defined as the physician's estimate that the patient will die within the next six months).
2. The patient has documented evidence of the progression of disease, such as X-ray findings or test results.

3. The patient has had either: (a) multiple hospitalizations or emergency room visits within the past six months, or (b) a documented decline in functional status (for homebound patients who have not been to a medical institution).

4. The patient and/or family has decided treatment aimed at curing the underlying disease is no longer appropriate.

5. The patient has diminished functional status as determined by meeting at least three of the following criteria:

   • Dependence on others for bathing
   • Dependence on others for dressing
   • Dependence on others for feeding
   • Dependence on others for moving from place to place (such as from bed to chair)
   • Incontinence of stool or urine
   • Inability to ambulate independently to the bathroom
   • Impaired nutritional status shown by: (a) intentional or progressive weight loss (more than 10 percent) over prior six months, or (b) low serum protein levels or low blood count

What to Expect from Hospice Care

Limitations of Hospice Care

Hospices offer important services to patients with advanced cancer and their families that are not available anywhere else, but there are some limitations to hospice care. Before enrolling in a hospice program, it is important to understand that, while they are staffed by sympathetic and caring people, most hospices in the United States are run like managed care organizations. This derives from the fact that when a person covered by Medicare enters a hospice program, Medicare stops paying for the person's other medical and hospital expenses. Instead, Medicare pays the hospice organization a per diem payment of approximately $100 for every day the patient spends in the hospice. The hospice organization is then responsible for paying for all expenses that otherwise would be covered by Medicare, such as hospital bills, lab tests, and doctor visits. Many hospices also provide the client's medications from this per diem amount.

When a hospice patient requires thousands of dollars of medical or hospital care, the hospice must pay those costs, but cannot pass any of them on to Medicare. Hospices are not high-profit businesses, so a few huge hospital bills could have a severe impact on the hospice's ability to provide other types of care, such as medication. Because of these financial constraints, the hospice limits what care it provides. These limitations should be made clear to you before you enter the program. However, the limitations of the hospice's care are likely to be the same as the patient's wishes for end of life care. For example, clients will no longer receive radiation or chemotherapy treatments and will not receive intensive care or "heroic" measures should complications develop.

It is important, however, to make certain that the limitations of care are acceptable before entering hospice. For example, some hospices may prevent a client from entering the hospital for almost any reason, or may actively try to prevent a client from making a visit to his original physician. Many physicians are reluctant to refer patients to a hospice because they feel, sometimes legitimately, that it may sever their relationship with a patient.

Benefits of Hospice Care

Some hospices are actual buildings that the patient stays in, but the overwhelming majority of American hospices provide at-home care for their clients, allowing them to spend their remaining days with family members. In fact, most hospices require the client to have either a full-time caregiver or a group of family members and friends that will take turns staying with her. There are few, if any, hospices that provide round-the-clock home care. Many hospices do, however, offer to provide patients with full-time care (often in a hospital or nursing home) for periods of up to five days to provide a rest for family members. If family members are not available to provide care, there may (or may not) be a hospice in your area that has a physical building where their clients can stay. As an alternative, many hospice services will provide care for people who are in nursing homes or other institutions.

There is a great deal of variability in the care provided by different hospice organizations. Some offer only basic nursing and counseling visits; others may have full-time physicians on staff and the ability to offer complex medical treatments at home. Most hospice clients are visited by a nurse several times a week and will be visited by other caregivers, such as nutritionists, home-health aides, physical therapists, and chaplains. Home hospice patients and their families also have access to around-the-clock telephone help and emergency visits.

More than 80 percent of clients entering a hospice program complain of pain. Hospice caregivers will help regulate pain medications to make sure a client is comfortable. Oral medications are used as much as possible, but most hospices can also give medication by injection or through continuous intravenous infusion. They may have access to advanced forms of pain therapy, such as patient-controlled intravenous pumps, but the use of these devices is discouraged in most hospices. Hospice caregivers also have expertise in treating other symptoms such as weakness, fatigue, shortness of breath, nausea, weight loss, and dry mouth.

One feature that differentiates hospice care from traditional medical care is the emphasis on family members actively participating in the care of the cancer patient. One of the primary aims of hospice care is the empowerment of family and friends so that they feel comfortable in providing this care. Under the guidance of hospice caregivers, family members undergo a de facto training program while caring for their loved one. It is not surprising that many hospice volunteers are family members of former hospice patients.

There is also great emphasis on relieving some of the psychological burdens that come with advanced cancer such as the distress of dying, the disruption of family and social ties, and the burden of being reliant on family and friends for physical care. Most hospices offer family members bereavement counseling and other supportive services for a year after the patient has died.

Summary

Hospice care is obviously not appropriate or desirable for everyone with terminal cancer. Many cancer patients, however, have spent so much time in hospitals that they prefer to spend their last months at home with family and friends. Hospice provides a way to achieve this while still receiving the medical care necessary to provide comfort and pain relief. It also provides psychological and emotional care that is rarely available in a hospital setting or medical practice.

Despite the proliferation of hospices and a growing acceptance of this type of care, only one-third of patients with advanced cancer ever receive hospice care, and most of those enter hospice during the last few weeks of their illness. There are potential barriers to entry into hospice care for patients with advanced cancer, ranging from a lack of insurance coverage to the emotional or physical inability of family members to participate in care. Many physicians are reluctant to refer patients to a hospice or are unwilling to "certify" that the patient will live for six months or less. (Most hospices allow for the recertification of patients who live beyond the six-month time span, however. The author has had cancer patients who have lived with hospice care for almost three years.) If hospice care sounds right for you, however, some resources to help you find a hospice in your area are listed in Appendix G.

Common Opioid Medications and Their Side Effects

Brand Name/Generic Name	Strength, Duration of Action

Butorphanol/Stadol — Weak to moderate, short acting

May cause withdrawal symptoms in individuals who have been taking other opioids

Most common side effects:
Constipation; drowsiness; lightheadedness; weakness; urinary retention.

Less common side effects:
Headache; dizziness; facial flushing; sweating; double vision; fever; indigestion; diarrhea; fainting; hallucinations; psychosis.

Codeine/Tylenol #3, Phenaphen #3 — Weak to moderate, short acting

Most common side effects:
Constipation; drowsiness; nausea.

Less common side effects:
Confusion; nausea or vomiting; excitement.

Fentanyl/Duragesic patches, Actiq lozenges — Potent, long acting

Most common side effects:
Drowsiness; lightheadedness; weakness; euphoria; dry mouth; urinary retention; constipation; slow or troubled breathing.

Less common side effects:
Allergic reactions; skin rash; dizziness; impaired concentration; confusion; depression; blurred or double vision; facial flushing; sweating; heart palpitation; nausea and vomiting.

Hydrocodone/Vicodin, Lorcet, Lortab   Weak to moderate, short acting
Most common side effects:
Constipation; drowsiness; dry mouth; urinary retention; light-headedness.
Less common side effects:
Allergic reactions; itching; dizziness; confusion; depression; nausea or vomiting; sweating; hallucinations; excitement.

Hydromorphone/Dilaudid   Potent, short acting
Most common side effects:
Anxiety; constipation; dizziness drowsiness; paranoia; urinary retention; nausea; vomiting; restlessness; sluggishness; sedation; troubled and slow breathing.
Less common side effects:
Agitation; blurred vision; chills; cramps; diarrhea; difficulty urinating; disorientation; double vision; dry mouth; depression; slow heartbeat; lightheadedness; hallucinations; loss of appetite; muscle rigidity; tremors; heart palpitations; sweating.

Levorphanol/Levo-Dromoran   Potent, long acting
Most common side effects:
Anxiety; constipation; dizziness; drowsiness; paranoia; urinary retention; nausea; vomiting; restlessness; sluggishness; sedation; troubled and slow breathing.
Less common side effects:
Blurred vision; cramps; diarrhea; difficulty urinating; disorientation; double vision; dry mouth; depression; slow heartbeat; faintness; flushing; headache.

Meperidine/Demerol, Mepergan   Moderate, short acting
Most common side effects:
Drowsiness; lightheadedness; weakness; euphoria; dry mouth; urinary retention; constipation; nausea.

Less common side effects:
Itching; headache; dizziness; confusion; depression; double vision; sweating; heart palpitation.

Methadone/Dolophine   Potent, long acting
Most common side effects:
Drowsiness; lightheadedness; weakness; euphoria; dry mouth; urinary retention; constipation; slow or troubled breathing.
Less common side effects:
Allergic reactions; headache; dizziness; impaired concentration; confusion; depression; blurred or double vision; sweating; heart palpitation; nausea and vomiting.

Opium/Tincture Opium 10%,
B & O suppositories   Potent, short acting
Most common side effects:
Drowsiness; lightheadedness; weakness; euphoria; dry mouth; urinary retention; constipation.
Less common side effects:
Allergic reactions; dizziness; confusion; depression; blurred or double vision; facial flushing; sweating; heart palpitation; nausea and vomiting.

Oxycodone/Percocet, Roxicodone   Potent, short acting, long acting in time-release form
Most common side effects:
Drowsiness; lightheadedness; dry mouth; urinary retention; constipation.
Less common side effects:
Allergic reactions; depression; blurred or double vision; nausea and vomiting.

Oxymorphone/Numorphan   Potent, short acting
Most common side effects:
Anxiety; constipation; dizziness; drowsiness; paranoia; urinary retention; nausea; restlessness; sluggishness; sedation.
Less common side effects:
Agitation; blurred vision; chills; cramps; double vision; dry mouth; depression; flushing; headache; insomnia; lightheadedness; loss of appetite; muscle

rigidity; tremors; heart palpitations; tingling or numbness; uncoordinated muscle movement.

Pentazocine/Talwin   Weak, short acting

May cause withdrawal symptoms in individuals who have been taking other opioids.

Most common side effects:

Constipation; drowsiness; lightheadedness; weakness; urinary retention.

Less common side effects:

Allergic reactions; facial flushing; sweating; blurred or double vision; nausea and vomiting; hypotension; hypertension; fever; indigestion; diarrhea.

Propoxyphene/Darvon   Weak, short acting

Most common side effects:

Drowsiness; dizziness; nausea; sedation.

Less common side effects:

Abdominal pain; constipation; euphoria; jaundice; kidney problems.

Generic and Brand Names of Nonopioid Medications Used for Pain Control

Nonsteroidal Anti-Inflammatory Drugs

Generic Name	Brand Names
Aspirin and caffeine	Vanquish, Excedrin, Excedrin X/S, Genaced, Goody's Headache, Anacin, As-Caff, Gensan, PAC Compound, Midol Max/Str, Midol PMS, BC Headache, Alka-Seltzer
Choline salicylate	Arthropan
Diclofenac potassium	Cataflam, Diclofenac, Voltaren
Diflunisal	Dolobid
Etodolac	Lodine
Fenoprofen calcium	Fenoprofen, Nalfon
Flurbiprofen	Ansaid, Flurbiprofen
Ibuprofen	Advil, BI Ibuprofen, Excedrin IB, Genpril, GNP Ibuprofen, Haltran, Ibuprofen, Menadol, Midol IB, Motrin, Motrin IB, Nuprin, Rufen
Indomethacin SA	Indocin, Indocin SR, Indomethacin
Ketoprofen	Ketoprofen, Orudis, Oruvail, Actron

Generic Name	Brand Names
Ketorolac tromethamine	Toradol
Meclofenamate sodium	Meclofenamate, Meclomen
Mefenamic acid	Asacol, Ponstel
Nabumetone	Relafen
Naproxen	Aleve, Naprosyn, Naproxen
Oxaprozin	Daypro
Piroxicam	Feldene
Salicylate	Tricolate, Trilisate
Salsalate	Salsalate, Disalcid, Salflex, Salicylsal AC
Sulindac	Clinoril, Sulindac
Tolmetin sodium	Tolectin, Tolectin DS, Tolmetin

Antiseizure Medications

Generic Name	Brand Names
Carbamazepine	Carbatrol, Tegretol, Epitol
Divalproex sodium	Depakote
Gabapentin	Neurontin
Lamotrigine	Lamictal
Oxcarbazepine	Trileptal
Tiagabine	Gabitril
Topiramate	Topamax
Valproate sodium	Depacon
Valproic acid	Depakene, Depakote
Vigabatrin	Sabril

Major Tranquilizers

Generic Name	Brand Names
Chlorpromazine	Thorazine
Clozapine	Clozaril
Droperidol	Inapsine

Fluphenazine	Prolixin, Fluphenaz, Permitil
Haloperidol	Haldol
Loxapine	Loxitane, Loxapine
Mesoridazine besylate	Serentil
Molindone	Moban
Perphenazine	Trilafon
Promazine	Sparine
Risperidone	Risperdal
Thioridazine	Mellaril, Thioridazine
Thiothixene	Navane
Trifluoperazine	Stelazine

Benzodiazepine Tranquilizers

Generic Name	Brand Names
Alprazolam	Xanax
Chlordiazepoxide	Librium
Clonazepam	Klonopin
Clorazepate	Tranxene
Diazepam	Valium, Dizac
Estazolam	Prosom
Flurazepam	Dalmane
Lorazepam	Ativan, Loraz
Oxazepam	Serax
Quazepam	Doral
Temazepam	Restoril
Triazolam	Halcion

Pain Treatment
Resources

Books like this can provide you with more complete information than any Internet site or educational pamphlet, but a book is always a year or so behind the newest technology. More recent information can often be found on the Internet. These days, if you don't have Internet access yourself, certainly someone you know does. If not, most local libraries have Internet terminals and are happy to show you how to use them.

You can find many sites by searching the Internet for the keywords "pain" and "cancer." When you go searching on your own, however, remember that the Internet is not regulated; anyone can claim almost anything they want. A lot of pages are infomercials for certain techniques, medications, or treatments. That doesn't mean they aren't reputable; the vast majority are. A site selling nutritional supplements can claim those supplements are the best thing in all of history. The Web site may look extremely professional and have a name that sounds like that of a major university or government site, such as the International University Consortium on Herbal Medicine. The reality may be that some guy pulled up grass out of his backyard, claimed it's an "ancient Oriental secret herbal all-natural cancer cure," set up an Internet site, and is selling it for $1,000 an ounce (people have already done just that; it's not a new idea). At best, it will take the government a year or two to close him down, if they can do it at all. To close him down, they have to prove in court that it's *not* a secret all-natural herbal cancer cure. That can be more difficult than it sounds.

If for no other reason than to save yourself hours scrolling through poor Internet sites or making wasted long-distance telephone calls, we recommend you start with some of the sites selected below. The organizations and Internet sites listed here are all reputable and give accurate information. They also provide links to other, equally reputable sites that may have more specific information about your disease. All the sites listed are useful, but we've placed *Best Site* next to the ones we recommend most highly as a place to start.

American Academy of Pain Management

http://www.aapm@aapainmanagement.org
13947 Mono Way, #A
Sonora, CA 95370
Tel: (209) 533-9744

A professional organization for physicians. It maintains a directory of pain treatment centers and pain management physicians.

American Alliance of Cancer Pain Initiatives

http://www.aacpi.org
1300 University Avenue, Suite 4720
Madison, WI 53706
Tel: (608) 265-4013
Fax: (608) 265-4014

An organization composed of the fifty state Cancer Pain Initiatives. These are voluntary organizations composed of medical professionals who promote cancer pain relief. They provide education, training, information, and organizational support to health care providers, cancer patients, and their families. The site is particularly good about the rules and regulations regarding controlled-substance treatment. It also publishes the *Cancer Pain Forum,* a newsletter.

American Pain Foundation

http://www.painfoundation@aol.com
111 South Calvert Street, Suite 2700
Baltimore, MD 21202

A good consumer site with links to pain treatment physicians, updates on pain management, and government rules and regulations.

American Pain Society

http://www.ampainsoc.org/links/patient.htm
4700 West Lake Avenue
Glenview, IL 60025
Tel: (847) 375-4715
Fax: (847) 375-4777

A research and medical practice and scientific organization. Its Web site has a directory of pain treatment centers and a large list of links to pain support groups.

American Cancer Society

Guidelines for Living with Cancer
http://www2.cancer.org/patientGuides/index.cfm

A nice listing of commonly asked questions about pain control, giving a lot of good advice and stopping a lot of myths about cancer pain. A place to start if you're feeling a bit overwhelmed by the "medicalese" of some other sites.

Cancer Care, Inc.   *Best Site*

http://www.info@cancercare.org
275 Seventh Avenue
New York, NY 10001
Tel: (212) 302-2400 or 1-800-813-HOPE (4673)
Fax: (212) 719-0263

A wonderful organization that provides many different types of support for cancer patients and their families. It publishes the *Helping Hand Resource Guide* to show what types of help are available for people with cancer and where you can find them. They also link to online and local support groups and have a lot of information on their site, including pain management and specific facts about the different types of cancer.

Cancer Resources from LifeCare Concepts

www.cancerresources.com
LifeCare Concepts
457 West 22nd Street, Suite B
New York, NY 10011
Tel: 1-800-401-2233

An organization dedicated exclusively to providing educational and support information for people living with cancer. It provides some educational material and videos, but the best resource is a well-organized Web site with links to many different information sources.

International Association for the Study of Pain

www.halcyon.com/iasp
IASP Secretariat
909 NE 43rd Street, Suite 306
Seattle, WA 98105-6020
Tel: (206) 547-6409
Fax: (206) 547-1703

Primarily focuses on research into pain and pain control. The site includes a newsflash feature and links to several current research groups' reports. Remember, though, a lot of this research is very preliminary and the treatments discussed may not be available for years.

Oncolink   *Best Site*

http://www.oncolink.com

A page maintained by the University of Pennsylvania Cancer Center. It has a lot of information about specific diseases and some information about pain management. Its recent news section is quite good. Its section on finances for cancer patients is unique and very helpful.

PAIN.COM   *Best Site*

http://www.pain.com/index.cfm

Dannemiller Memorial Educational Foundation

Possibly the best medical site on the Internet on any topic. This site is run by an extremely reputable nonprofit company whose sole purpose is to provide education for health care professionals. PAIN.COM is supported by grants from several large medical companies, but there is no editorializing of its products and only minimal advertising. Although the site contains a massive amount of material for both physicians and patients, it is so clearly organized that anyone can navigate it very quickly. Start here. Chances are, if it doesn't have the information you want, one of its links will.

Partners Against Pain

http://www.partnersagainstpain.com/

Sponsored by a manufacturer of pain control medications, it not surprisingly has a bit of self-serving public relations. It does, however, maintain a nice set of current links to cancer pain sites.

Talaria

http://www.statsci.com/talaria/talaria.html

A site geared to physicians who treat pain. Not as easy to navigate or as readily understandable as some sites. It does have a lot of specific information about pain control measures and an online textbook about cancer pain that's easy to read.

World Health Organization

Cancer Pain Guidelines

http://www.medsch.wisc.edu/WHOcancerpain/

The site allows you to request copies of the quarterly World Health Organization reports on cancer pain management.

Cancer
Support Groups

Your oncologist probably has already put you in touch with local cancer support groups or referred you to a counselor. If not, there are so many different support groups that you may get lost trying to find the services you would like. This list focuses on groups that provide emotional support and education. It contains organizations that provide everything from one-on-one support from a cancer survivor volunteer, to local support groups, to Internet chat rooms, and even national meetings. Most also offer educational material either on their Web site or in booklets that they will happily send you at no cost. We've placed *Best Site* next to the ones we recommend most highly as a place to start.

General Cancer Support Groups

American Cancer Society
http://www.cancer.org
Tel: 1-800-118-2345

Operates an informational Web page with separate sections on adult and pediatric brain tumors, provides written booklets, and offers advice and help through the 800 number listed. The ACS also supports research, provides printed materials, and conducts educational programs. A local ACS unit may be listed in your telephone directory under "American Cancer Society."

American Institute for Cancer Research (AICR)

http://www.aicr.org
1759 R Street, NW
Washington, DC 20009
Tel: (202) 328-7744 or 1-800-843-8114

Despite its name, this isn't really a research site, although the organization does fund cancer research. The AICR provides information about cancer prevention, particularly through diet and nutrition. It has a pen pal support network and brochures about diet and nutrition.

CancerNet from the National Cancer Institute   *Best Site*

http://www.cancernet.nci.nih.gov/index.html

One of the best government sites around. This large, well-organized site provides a lot of educational information and links to support groups, research sites and clinical trials, and a host of other useful things. You can also order much of its information to be sent to you free of charge.

Cancer Care   *Best Site*

http://www.info@cancercare.org
275 Seventh Avenue
New York, NY 10001
Tel: (212) 302-2400 or 1-800-813-HOPE (4673)
Fax: (212) 719-0263

Provides free, professional assistance to people with any type of cancer, at any stage of illness, and to their families. Offers education, one-on-one counseling, specialized support groups, financial assistance for nonmedical expenses, home visits by trained volunteers, and referrals to community services. A section of the Cancer Care Web site and some publications are available in Spanish, and staff can respond to calls and E-mails in Spanish.

CancerGuide
http://www.cancerguide.org

A private page set up by the spouse of a cancer victim. Usually, we do not recommend such sites because they tend not to be informative, but this one is excellent. It is particularly appropriate if you are starting on a research quest to learn about cancer. It not only has lots of useful links, but also instructional sections on exactly how to research a certain type of cancer, which could save you lots of time.

Cancer Hope Network
http://www.cancerhopenetwork.org
Two North Road, Suite A
Chester, NJ 07930
Tel: 1-877-HOPENET (1-877-467-3638)

Cancer Hope Network provides individual support to cancer patients and their families by matching them with trained volunteers who have undergone and recovered from a similar cancer experience. This service is also available in Spanish.

Cancer Internet Discussion Group
Alt.Support.cancer

This site can be a great way to meet people who've been there and get practical advice and information. Remember, though, it's a freelance discussion group. Anyone can say anything, and sometimes they do. If you've never participated in an Internet discussion group, or don't know how to sign in, information is available through the FAQ sheet.

Cancer Studies for Determined People
http://www.mother.com/~wesurviv/welcome.htm

Another site of the type we rarely recommend, set up by a cancer survivor. The site contains *a lot* of "alternative medicine" information. Some of the information is good, but some is the worst kind of pseudo-science. It does, however, contain some excellent information on psychology and support groups for cancer patients and offers some direct support services.

Gilda's Club

http://www.gildasclub.org
195 West Houston Street
New York, NY 10014
Tel: (212) 647-9700

The club provides social and emotional support to cancer patients, their families, and friends. Lectures, workshops, networking groups, special events, and a children's program are available.

National Cancer Institute

http://cis.nci.nih.gov/
Tel: 1-800-4-CANCER (1-800-422-6237)
TTY: 1-800-332-8615

Provides updates on new research and operates a cancer information service. The same information can be found in an easier to navigate format at CancerNet, which is a National Cancer Institute Web site. The telephone service, however, provides information specialists who can help translate the latest scientific information into understandable language (English, Spanish, or on TTY equipment).

National Coalition for Cancer Survivorship (NCCS)

http://www.cansearch.org
1010 Wayne Avenue, Suite 505
Silver Spring, MD 20910-5600
Tel: (301) 650-8868 or 1-888-YES-NCCS (1-888-650-9127)

A network of groups and individuals that offer support to cancer survivors and their loved ones. Provides information and resources on cancer support, advocacy, and quality-of-life issues. A section of the NCCS Web site and a limited selection of publications are available in Spanish.

Oncolink

http://www.oncolink.com

A page maintained by the University of Pennsylvania Cancer Center. It has a lot of information about specific diseases and some information about pain management. It has a recent news section that is quite good. Its section on finances for cancer patients is unique and very helpful.

R. A. Bloch Cancer Foundation

http://www.blochcancer.org
4435 Main Street, Suite 500
Kansas City, MO 64111
Tel: (816) 932-8453 or 1-800-433-0464

Matches newly diagnosed cancer patients with trained, home-based volunteers who have been treated for the same type of cancer. Also distributes informational materials, including a multidisciplinary list of institutions that offer second opinions.

Vital Options and "The Group Room" Cancer Radio Talk Show

http://www.vitaloptions.org
P.O. Box 19233
Encino, CA 91416-9233
Tel: (818) 508-5657 or 1-800-GRP-ROOM (1-800-477-7666)
(Sundays, 4 P.M. to 6 P.M. EST)

A weekly syndicated call-in cancer talk show linking callers with other patients, long-term survivors, family members, physicians, and therapists experienced in working with and discussing cancer issues.

The Wellness Community

http://www.wellness-community.org
35 East Seventh Street, Suite 412
Cincinnati, OH 45202
Tel: (513) 421-7111 or 1-888-793-WELL (1-888-793-9355)

Provides free psychological and emotional support to cancer patients and their families. Offers support groups facilitated by licensed therapists, stress reduction and cancer education workshops, nutrition guidance, exercise sessions, and social events.

Support Resources for Families of Childhood Cancer Victims

Candlelighters Childhood Cancer Foundation
http://www.candle.org
7910 Woodmont Avenue, Suite 460
Bethesda, MD 20814
Tel: (301) 657-8401 or 1-800-366-2223
Fax: (301) 718-2686

A nonprofit organization that offers services for all family members of childhood cancer victims. Provides information, peer support, over four hundred publications, an information clearinghouse, and a network of local support groups. A financial aid list provides organizations to which eligible families may apply for assistance.

The Compassionate Friends
http://www.compassionatefriends.org/
Tel: (630) 990-0010

This wonderful organization exists only to help grieving parents cope with the loss of a child. It has chapters in every state and throughout Canada.

National Childhood Cancer Foundation (NCCF)
http://www.nccf.org
440 East Huntington Drive
P.O. Box 60012
Arcadia, CA 91066-6012
Tel: (626) 447-1674, ext. 198 or 1-800-458-6223

Supports research conducted by a network of institutions, each of which has a team of doctors, scientists, and other specialists in the diagnosis, treatment, supportive care, and research on the cancers of infants, children, and young adults. Advocating for children with cancer and the centers that treat them is also a focus.

Support Resources for Specific Types of Cancer

Brain Cancer

American Brain Tumor Association (ABTA)
http://www.abta.org
2720 River Road, Suite 146
Des Plaines, IL 60018
Tel: (847) 827-9910 or 1-800-886-ABTA (1-800-886-2282)

Provides educational information including printed and online materials about research and treatment of brain tumors. Also provides listings of physicians, treatment facilities, and support groups throughout the country. A limited selection of Spanish-language publications is available.

National Brain Tumor Foundation (NBTF)
http://www.braintumor.org
414 Thirteenth Street, Suite 700
Oakland, CA 94612
Tel: (510) 839-9777 or 1-800-934-CURE (1-800-934-2873)

Publishes printed materials for patients and family members, provides access to a national network of patient support groups, and assists in answering patient inquiries. Staff are available to answer calls in either English or Spanish, and there are some Spanish-language publications available.

Breast Cancer

ENCORE
http://www.ywca.org
YWCA of the USA
Office of Women's Health Advocacy
624 Ninth Street, NW, Third Floor
Washington, DC 20001-5303
Tel: (202) 628-3636 or 1-800-95E-PLUS (1-800-953-7587)

ENCORE is the YWCA's discussion and exercise program for women who have had breast cancer surgery. Your local branch of the YWCA can provide more information about ENCORE.

National Alliance of Breast Cancer Organizations (NABCO)
http://www.nabco.org
9 East 37th Street, 10th Floor
New York, NY 10016
Tel: (212) 889-0606 or 1-888-80-NABCO (1-888-806-2226)

Although focused on legislative concerns of breast cancer patients, NABCO also provides educational material about breast cancer and maintains a list, organized by state, of support groups.

Y-ME National Breast Cancer Organization
http://www.y-me.org
212 West Van Buren Street
Chicago, IL 60607-3908
Tel: (312) 986-8338 or 1-800-221-2141 (English) or
1-800-986-9505 (Spanish)

Provides a national hotline, organizes early detection workshops, and has support programs run through local chapter offices throughout the United States.

Kidney/Renal Cancer

Kidney Cancer Association
http://www.nkca.org
1234 Sherman Avenue, Suite 203
Evanston, IL 60202-1375
Tel: (847) 332-1051 or 1-800-850-9132

Offers printed materials about the diagnosis and treatment of kidney cancer, sponsors support groups, and provides physician referral information.

Lymphoma/Leukemia

Cure For Lymphoma Foundation (CFL)
http://www.cfl.org
215 Lexington Avenue
New York, NY 10016-6023
Tel: (212) 213-9595 or 1-800-CFL-6848 (1-800-235-6848)

Offers support and education programs, booklets, family forums, teleconferences, support groups, and a monthly newsletter. It also has a nationwide Patient-to-Patient Telephone Network and networking groups and a toll-free information line.

Lymphoma Research Foundation of America (LRFA)

http://www.lymphoma.org
8800 Venice Boulevard, Suite 207
Los Angeles, CA 90034
Tel: (310) 204-7040 or 1-800-500-9976

Provides educational information and has a helpline for general information. It has support groups and a buddy program matching newly diagnosed patients with other lymphoma patients who have coped with the disease. It will also help with referrals to oncologists, clinical trials, and support groups.

Leukemia Society of America (LSA)

http://www.leukemia.org
600 Third Avenue, Fourth Floor
New York, NY 10016
Tel: (212) 573-8484 or 1-800-955-4LSA (1-800-955-4572)

Offers services to patients with leukemia, lymphoma, Hodgkin's disease, and multiple myeloma. Provides health education materials and a supervised peer support program. It also makes referrals and in some cases offers financial aid for certain treatment and transportation expenses.

Lung Cancer

Alliance for Lung Cancer Advocacy, Support, and Education (ALCASE)

http://www.alcase.org
1601 Lincoln Avenue
Vancouver, WA 98660
Tel: (360) 696-2436 or 1-800-298-2436

Provides education programs and psychosocial support for lung cancer victims and their families, and advocacy about issues concerning lung cancer survivors.

Multiple Myeloma

International Myeloma Foundation (IMF)

http://www.myeloma.org
2129 Stanley Hills Drive
Los Angeles, CA 90046
Tel: (323) 654-3023 or 1-800-452-CURE (1-800-452-2873)

Provides a toll-free hotline, seminars, and educational materials for patients and their families. Keeps a list of other organizations' support groups and provides information on how to start a support group.

Multiple Myeloma Research Foundation (MMRF)

http://www.multiplemyeloma.org
11 Forest Street
New Canaan, CT 06840
Tel: (203) 972-1250

Publishes a quarterly newsletter and provides referrals and information packets free of charge to patients and family members.

Ovarian Cancer

National Ovarian Cancer Coalition (NOCC)

http://www.ovarian.org
2335 East Atlantic Boulevard, Suite 401
Pompano Beach, FL 33062
Tel: (954) 781-3500 or 1-888-OVARIAN (1-888-682-7426)

Has a toll-free telephone number for information, referral, support, and education about ovarian cancer. Also offers support groups and has a database of gynecologic oncologists searchable by state.

Ovarian Cancer National Alliance

http://www.ovariancancer.org
1627 K Street, 12th Floor
Washington, DC 20006
Tel: (202) 331-1332

Distributes informational materials, sponsors an annual advocacy conference for survivors, and works with women's groups, seniors, and health professionals to increase awareness of ovarian cancer.

Prostate Cancer

US TOO International

http://www.ustoo.com
930 North York Road, Suite 50
Hinsdale, IL 60521
Tel: (630) 323-1002 or 1-800-80-US-TOO (1-800-808-7866)

A prostate cancer support group organization offering educational materials, support groups, and new information about treatment for this disease.

Other Useful Resources

Help in Obtaining Treatments
If Your Insurance Has Denied

The National Guideline Clearing House

http://www.guideline.gov/index.asp

This site, although a dry government site that can be a bit difficult to navigate, allows you to download practice guidelines developed by different medical organizations. The guidelines may force an insurer to provide treatment it has claimed is "not standard" or "experimental."

Patient Advocate Foundation (PAF)

http://www.patientadvocate.org

780 Pilot House Drive, Suite 100-C

Newport News, VA 23606

Tel: (757) 873-6668 or 1-800-532-5274

Provides education, legal counseling, and referrals to cancer patients and survivors concerning managed care, insurance, financial issues, job discrimination, and debt crisis matters.

Other Services

National Lymphedema Network (NLN)
http://www.lymphnet.org
2211 Post Street, Suite 404
San Francisco, CA 94115-3427
Tel: (415) 921-1306 or 1-800-541-3259

Provides education and guidance to patients suffering from lymphedema following cancer surgery and treatment. Provides a toll-free support hotline, a referral service to lymphedema treatment centers, a quarterly newsletter, support groups, and pen pals.

National Marrow Donor Program
http://www.marrow.org
3433 Broadway Street, NE, Suite 500
Minneapolis, MN 55413
Tel: (612) 627-5800 or 1-800-MARROW-2 (1-800-627-7692)

Funded by the federal government, the program keeps a registry of potential bone marrow donors and provides free information on bone marrow transplantation, peripheral blood stem cell transplant, cord blood transplants, and unrelated donor stem cell transplant.

The United Ostomy Association, Inc.
http://www.uoa.org
19772 MacArthur Boulevard, Suite 200
Irvine, CA 92612-2405
Tel: (949) 660-8624 or 1-800-826-0826 (7:30 A.M.–4:30 P.M. PT)

Helps ostomy patients by providing mutual aid and emotional support. Provides information to patients and the public and sends volunteers to visit with new ostomy patients.

Finding Information on Cancer Studies and Research Trials

Your doctor can be a great resource for finding research programs and clinical trials that are appropriate for you, but he can't keep up with every research program that's available. If you are truly interested in participating in a research study, you may have to investigate it yourself. Most research programs last less than a year, so keeping current is important. For that reason, Internet sites are usually the best way to get the information you need.

Cancer Trials
http://cancertrials.nci.nih.gov/

CenterWatch
http://www.centerwatch.com/
This organization maintains a general database of all types of clinical research trials. There are a fair number of cancer and pain management clinical trials, and the site has a search feature so you can find them. You can also sign up to be notified by E-mail whenever a new clinical trial for your cancer is added to the database.

Oncolink Clinical Trials Registry
http://cancer.med.upenn.edu/clinical_trials/
The Oncolink Web site is recommended in almost every one of the appendixes, and its subsection on clinical trials is no exception. It is

excellent, offering access not only to government-sponsored, but also to private research studies.

Southwest Oncology Group Clinical Trials

http://www.oo.saci.org

This is one of several major cooperative cancer research groups in the United States that conducts numerous clinical trials. The Web site contains an index of clinical trials it is participating in, but the entries are very brief. If one of the studies sounds appropriate, you can contact the group directly, or ask your doctor to contact them.

UKCCCR Clinical Trials Registry

http://www.cto.mrc.ac.uk/ukcccr/

This is a database of British clinical trials and has a sophisticated search engine. This database tends to list many trials that have already finished accruing patients—be sure to use the "Status/Centres" option to limit the search to open trials. Many of the trials will accept non–United Kingdom citizens, although you would have to travel there at your own expense.

Radiation Therapy Oncology Group (RTOG)

http://www.rtog.org/

This national cooperative research organization operates under the auspices of the American College of Radiology. It conducts multicenter clinical trials, usually combining surgery, radiation, and chemotherapy in attempts to improve long-term cancer treatment outcomes.

The International Oncology Study Group (IOSG)

http://www.iosg.org
4515 Verone
Bellaire, TX 77401
Tel: (713) 432-7229

This is a cooperative research group similar to Southwest Oncology Group, that conducts clinical studies to improve the prognosis for patients with cancer.

Resources for Hospice Care

Hospice Services

Children's Hospice International
http://www.chionline.org
2202 Mount Vernon Avenue, Suite 3C
Alexandria, VA 22301
Tel: (703) 684-0330 or 1-800-2-4-CHILD (1-800-242-4453)

Provides a network of support for dying children and their families. It has support groups and offers educational materials and training programs for pain management and care of seriously ill children.

Hospice Education Institute/Hospicelink
190 Westbrook Road
Essex, CT 06426
Tel: (860) 767-1620 or 1-800-331-1620
E-mail: hospiceall@aol.com

Provides some information and referral services and advice regarding hospice and palliative care.

Hospice Link
http://www.hospiceworld.org
Hospice Education Institute
190 Westbrook Road
Essex, CT 06426-1510
Tel: (860) 767-1620 or 1-800-331-1620

Hospice Link helps patients and their families find support services in their communities. Offers information about hospice and can refer cancer patients and their families to local hospice programs.

National Hospice Organization (NHO)   *Best Site*
http://www.nho.org
1901 North Moore Street, Suite 901
Arlington, VA 22209-1714
Tel: (703) 243-5900 or 1-800-658-8898

An association of groups that provide hospice care. Offers discussion groups, publications, information about how to find a hospice, and information about the financial aspects of hospice.

National Association for Home Care
http://www.nahc.org/
c/o Consumer Guide
P.O. Box 14241
Washington, DC 20003
Tel: (202) 547-7424

This site is a trade association, but it can provide referrals to local hospice organizations.

National Institute for Jewish Hospice
8723 Alden Drive, Suite 219
Los Angeles, CA 90048
Tel: (310) 854-3036 or 1-800-446-4448

Provides free telephone counseling and referrals specifically for terminally ill Jewish patients.

Related Services

Last Acts

www.lastacts.org

A national organization devoted to improving the quality of care at the end of life. It not only concerns itself with medical care, but also has wonderful articles about how family and patients can cope with the last stages of life, and practical advice. The site is currently very slow to download, however.

Choice in Dying

www.choices.org
1035 Thirtieth Street NW
Washington, DC 20007
Tel: (202) 338-9790

A group dedicated to the advocacy for the rights of terminally ill persons. Provides information about complex end-of-life decisions, such as living wills and advance directives. Provides some counseling for patients and families and offers a range of publications and services.

Selected References

Textbooks

Arbit, E., ed. 1993. *Management of Cancer-Related Pain*. Armonk, NY: Futura.

Joy, J. E. et al, eds. 1999. The Medical Value of Marijuana and Related Substances. Chap. 4 in *Marijuana and Medicine: Assessing the Science Base*. Washington, D.C.: National Academy Press.

Kübler-Ross, E. 1997. *On Death and Dying*. New York: Simon & Schuster.

McGuire, D. B. et al. 1995 *Cancer Pain Management,* 2d edition. Sudbury, MA: Jones and Bartlett.

Parris, W. C. 1996. *Cancer Pain Management: Principles and Practice*. Woburn, MA: Butterworth-Heinemann.

Patt, R. B. 1992. *Cancer Pain*. New York: Lippincott-Raven.

Medical Journal Articles

American Society of Anesthesiology. 1996. Practice guidelines for cancer pain management. *Anesthesiology* 1243–57.

Calissi, P. T., and L. A. Jaber. 1995. Peripheral diabetic neuropathy: Current concepts in treatment. *The Annals of Pharmacotherapy* 29: 769–77.

Chabal, C. et al. 1997. Prescription opiate abuse in chronic pain patients: Clinical criteria, incidence, and predictors. *Clinical Journal of Pain* 13:150–55.

Cryer, B., and M. Feldman. 1998. Cyclooxygenase-1 and cyclooxygenase-2 selectivity of widely used nonsteroidal anti-inflammatory drugs. *American Journal of Medicine* 104(5):413–21.

Derby, S. A. 1999. Opioid conversion guidelines for managing adult cancer pain." *American Journal of Nursing* 62–65.

Godfrey, R. G. 1996. A guide to the understanding and use of tricyclic antidepressants in the overall management of fibromyalgia and other chronic pain syndromes. *Archives of Internal Medicine* 156:1047–52.

Karlsten, R., and T. Gordh. 1997. How do drugs relieve neurogenic pain? *Drugs & Aging* 11:398–412.

Kingery, W. S. 1997. A critical review of controlled clinical trials for peripheral neuropathic pain and complex regional pain syndromes. *Pain* 73:123–39.

Kori, H. et al. 1997. Clinical practice guidelines: Management of bone pain secondary to metastatic disease. *Journal of the Moffitt Cancer Center* 4(2):153–57.

Lipman, A. G. 1996. Analgesic drugs for neuropathic and sympathetically maintained pain. *Clinical Geriatric Medicine* 12:501–15.

Majeroni, B. et al. 1998. The pharmacologic treatment of depression. *American Board of Family Practice* 11(2):127–39.

McQuay, H. J. et al. 1996. A systematic review of antidepressants in neuropathic pain. *Pain* 68:217–27.

Mercadante, S. 1999. Cancer control special report: World Health Organization guidelines: Problem areas in cancer pain management. *Journal of the Moffitt Cancer Center* 6(2):191–97.

———. 1999. Opioid rotation for cancer pain: Rationale and clinical aspects. *Cancer* 86(9):1856–66.

Merskey, H. 1997. Pharmacological approaches other than opioids in chronic non-cancer pain management. *Acta Anaesthesiologica Scandinavica* 41:187–90.

Ollat, H., and P. Cesaro. 1995. Pharmacology of neuropathic pain. *Clinical Neuropharmacology* 18:391–404.

Portenoy, R. K. 1999. Management of cancer pain. *Lancet* 353: 1695–700.

Vigano, A. 1996. Individualized use of methadone and opioid rotation in the comprehensive management of cancer pain associated with poor prognostic indicators. *Pain* 67(1):115–19.

Wetzel, C. H., and J. F. Connelly. 1997. Use of gabapentin in pain management. *The Annals of Pharmacotherapy* 31:1082–3.

Zakrzewska, J. M. et al. 1997. Lamotrigine (lamictal) in refractory trigeminal neuralgia: Results from a double-blind placebo controlled crossover trial. *Pain* 73:223–30.

Index

Page references followed by the letter *t* indicate tabular material.

Spinoreticular tract, 12
Spinothalamic tract, 12, 188, 189
SSAs. *See* Serotonin specific
    antidepressants
SSRIs. *See* Selective serotonin reup-
    take inhibitors
St. John's wort (hypericum), 157,
    158
Stadol (butorphanol), 101, 133–34,
    245
Stellate ganglion nerve blocks,
    182–83
Steroid pseudorheumatism, 48
Steroids. *See* Corticosteroids
Stimulants, 62t, 66, 121
Stomach
    obstruction of, 30
    problems with NSAIDS, 105–7
Stress, 6, 51
Strokes, 32
Strontium-89 treatment, 210–11
Subcutaneous catheters, 137–38
Subdural injections, 175, 177–78
Sublingual tablets, 134
Suffering *vs.* pain, 4–6
Sulindac, 110
Superior hypogastric plexus block,
    178–79, 187
Superior vena cava syndrome, 33,
    146
Support groups, 60–61, 166,
    259–69
Suppositories, 131–32, 247
Surgery
    incisional and postoperative pain,
        39–40
    pain associated with, 37–38
    palliative, 38

postoperative syndromes, 40–42,
    216–18
Swelling
    controlling with corticosteroids,
        48
    in lymphedema, 33
    side effect of opioids, 99
    from tumors infiltrating into
        nerves, 214–15
Sympathectomy, surgical, 219
Sympathetic nerve blocks
    bier, 183–84
    indications for, 174
    lumbar sympathetic, 181–82
    other blocks near spine, 177–79
    stellate ganglion, 182–83
Sympathetic nervous system, 19–20,
    218–19
Sympathetically mediated pain,
    19–20
    nerve blocks for, 181–84
    treatment of, 218–19
Symptoms. *See also specific symptoms*
    antidepressants for, 63t
    of anxiety, 67
    associated with pain, 85
    of depression, 59–60
    keeping diary of, 83–84
Synapses, 10–11

T
Talwin (pentazocine), 101, 248
TCAs. *See* Tricyclic antidepressants
Tea, green, 163
Tegretol (carbamazepine), 116
TENS (transcutaneous electrical
    nerve stimulation), 171
Thalamus, 13